ILLUSTRATED GUIDE TO

TAPING TECHNIQUES

Karin A. Austin
B.P.T., B.Sc. (P.T.)

Consultant Physiotherapist
Physiotherapie Internationale K.A.Inc.
and
L'Esprit Sport Rehabilitation

Kathryn A. Gwynn-Brett
B.Sc. (P.T.)

Sole Charge Physiotherapist
Mississauga Orthopaedic and Sports Injury Clinic

Sarah C. Marshall
B.Sc. (P.T.)

Clinical Coordinator and Staff Physiotherapist
Ste-Anne's Hospital
Faculty Lecturer
McGill University

Mosby-Wolfe

London Baltimore Bogotá Boston Buenos Aires Caracas Carlsbad, CA Chicago
Madrid Mexico City Milan Naples, FL New York Philadelphia St. Louis Sydney Tokyo Toronto Wiesbaden

Copyright © 1994 Mosby-Year Book Europe Limited
Published in 1994 by Wolfe Publishing, an imprint of
Times Mirror International Publishers Ltd.
Printed by BPC Hazell Books Ltd
ISBN 0 7234 1635 4

Reprinted in 1996.

For full details of all Times Mirror International Publishers Limited titles please
write to Times Mirror International Publishers Limited, Lynton House, 7–12
Tavistock Square, London. WC1H 9LB.

A CIP catalogue record for this book is available from the British Library.

PREFACE

The Illustrated Guide to Taping Techniques is appropriate for use as:

* *a textbook in sports medicine and physiotherapy courses*
* *a manual for sports coaches*
* *a guide for emergency room staff*
* *a source of specific reference material for sports clinics, treatment centres or for any setting where injuries requiring taping support are encountered.*

Uniquely designed to accommodate the requirements of clinicians as well as sports personnel, this guide offers highly informative, clearly illustrated taping methods developed by persons actively involved in physiotherapy and in sports medicine. The authors' collective experience involves multiple aspects of these fields including teaching, clinical application, and active involvement as medical support personnel at Olympic Games.

An authoritative, comprehensive guide, **The Illustrated Guide to Taping Techniques** will prove indispensable to students of medicine, physiotherapy and athletic therapy as well as being instructive to those involved with athletes: coaches, trainers, physical educators, managers, the athletes themselves and their families. It is recommended both as a teaching manual, as well as a practical guide in hospital emergency rooms, sports clinics, physiotherapy centres and on site at athletic events.

Crucial to effective treatment of injuries requiring taping are an understanding of the type and degree of injury, the tissues involved, the taping material best suited to the situation and the proper application of those materials. Referring to this guide, the treatment person will be able to handle complex situations by using the appropriate, effective taping techniques for providing adequate compression, stability and support to the injured structure. Whether the desired effect is immediate return to athletic participation or gradual rehabilitation, once the injury has been properly assessed, correct application of the specific taping technique to the injured area will ensure maximum protection and mobility.

This guide has been organised into two distinct divisions, the first covers taping supplies with a general description of their characteristics and uses; principles of taping including basic taping guidelines with a unique review system using the acronyms **S.U.P.P.O.R.T.** and **P.R.E.C.A.U.T.I.O.N.**; charts for sprains, strains, and contusions using the mnemonic **T.E.S.T.S.**, plus an overview of various types of tape strips.

The second section covers precise taping techniques for specific injuries. Clear step-by-step photographs and detailed instructions guide the taper. A list of supplies and positioning relative to each taping application is included, and a sample injury assessment and treatment chart follows each technique.

Once the information in this guide has been assimilated and the techniques have been mastered, the taper will have acquired an excellent base. Professionals involved in the taping of sports-related injuries will, through experience, develop the ability to adapt the principles and techniques described in this guide to an infinite number of situations.

CONTENTS ···

···

ACKNOWLDGEMENTS

The authors would like to thank the following people and corporations for their assistance in completing this project.

Janet Adams, Montreal, who edited, restructured and helped revise the final book and without whose help this end product would not have been possible.

Dr Tracy Cooper, Commissioning Editor, Mosby Year Book Europe, for her patience and continued faith in our project.

Patrick Daly, former Editor, Mosby Year Book Europe, for initiating the project.

Mosby Year Book Europe, for providing financial assistance.

Wendy Dayton, Montreal for her initial editorial assistance.

Debbie Jamroz and **Aubert Brillant,** THE PROFESSIONALS PHOTO STUDIO, Montreal, Quebec, whose expertise and patience produced the excellent photographs of our technique.

Judith Martin and **Carlos Ramirez,** the models who put up with long hours under hot lights in cold studios.

Smith & Nephew Inc., whose generous grant and donation of taping supplies enabled us to proceed.

Woodward & Sons Ltd., who provided additional taping materials.

NDG PHOTO, Montreal, Quebec, who provided preliminary photography equipment.

The many experienced therapists who, over the years, have shared their techniques and knowledge, allowing us to learn and to develop and improve skills that can now be offered to others.

Finally, to our families whose patience and understanding bolstered our spirits and heightened our resolve during the long hours involved in bringing this book to its finished form, heartfelt thanks to all.

Chapter One ....

TAPING SUPPLIES

Any successful taping job begins with choosing quality materials. Top quality tape is more reliable and consistent than poor quality tape and is essential if optimal protection is to be achieved. Tape quality affects the degree of compression, stability and support necessary for a properly executed taping technique.

Included in this chapter are descriptions of and uses for various taping supplies. These supplies have been divided into three lists. The bare essentials for taping are included in the first list. Additional essential items necessary for a field kit are grouped in the second list. The optional supplies in the third list should also be available but are not mandatory. Many more items could be added to a well equipped taping kit – but we have covered only the most important supplies.

ESSENTIAL SUPPLIES: DESCRIPTION.

Adhesive elastic tape: Elastoplast™
This tape offers elasticity as well as adhesion. Useful for a wide range of purposes:
- maintaining localized compression over a contusion
- keeping maximal pressure on a sprain
- forming an "anchor" around a muscle area
- keeping a brace in place.

Quality characteristics:
- strong recoil. To test, stretch an 80 cm (32 in.) strip to maximum length. Hold for 30 seconds, then release. Tape should return to 125% of original length (100 cm; 40 in.).
- the roll should be encased in airtight wrapping.

Inferior:
- little or no recoil.
- tendency to unravel at the edges.
- does not adhere well; tends to peel off easily.

Antiseptic lotion; antibiotic ointment; antifungal spray or powder
- useful as a secondary precaution in treating minor abrasions, blisters, lacerations and tape cuts
- apply to cleaned wounds prior to taping
- use sparingly so as not to interfere with the adhesive properties of the overall tape job.

ESSENTIAL TAPING SUPPLIES:
razor and soap
skin toughener spray
lubricating ointment
heel and lace pads
underwrap
white zinc oxide tape 3.8 cm (1.5 in.) width
adhesive elastic tape 7.5 cm (3 in.)
bandage scissors
padding: felt or foam
elastic bandages (7.5 cm) (3 in.), (15 cm) (6 in.)

ADDITIONAL ITEMS FOR FIELD KIT:
antiseptic solution
cotton gauze squares: sterile and non-sterile
plastic band aid strips
triangular bandages
ice and towels
pen, pencil and paper
exact change for telephone

OPTIONAL SUPPLIES:
surgical gloves
instant cold packs
antibiotic ointment
antifungal spray or powder
blister protectors
cotton-tipped applicators
tongue depressors
quick drying adhesive spray
waterproof tape
white zinc oxide tape 1.2 cm (0.5 in.) width
white zinc oxide tape 5 cm (2 in.)
elastic adhesive tape 3.8 cm (1.5 in.)
adhesive remover
tape cutters
nail clippers; nail scissors

White zinc oxide tape: 3.8 cm (1.5 in.)

The basic all-purpose tape essential to any taping kit used in any sport. Adhesive, non-elastic and available in rolls of various lengths, white zinc oxide tape is indispensable.

Quality characteristics:

- slightly porous to permit some lateral glide or stretch (shearing) across the bias of the tape.
- To test: grasp a 5 cm (2 in.) piece of tape between your two hands and pull laterally. The tape should shear about 20° in either direction without creasing (as in the photographs below).

Inferior:

- when tested as described above, a poor grade of tape will start to crease and to stick together almost as soon as any sideways stress is induced. Other types of inexpensive tape may have two or more lengths stitched end to end. Although the quality may not be inferior, it will not give a smooth, uniform look to the taping job. Any seams must be cut away before applying the tape.

> NOTE:
> All types of tape should be kept in a cool, dry place. Rotate supplies to ensure freshness: old tape gets too sticky.

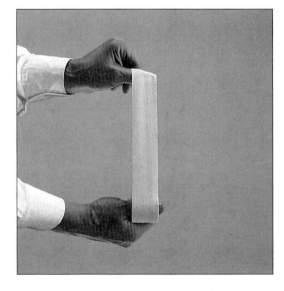
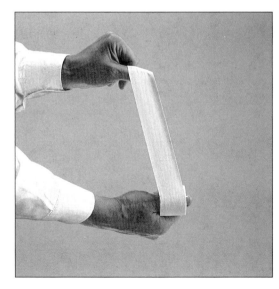
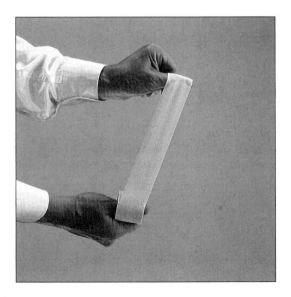

Skin toughener spray: Tuff-Skin™; Skin Tuffner™

- fast-drying aerosol sprays forming a microscopic adhesive layer protecting skin from contact with tape irritants
- provides an additional adhesive layer

Quality characteristics:
- dries quickly
- adheres well

Inferior:
- can irritate sensitive skin
- difficult to remove

> TIP: Some brands are less apt to cause irritation in specific chemical-sensitive athletes. Having several brands on hand will enable tape-applier to try alternatives with different chemical ingredients.

Adhesive spray: Q.D.A.™

- quick-drying adhesive sprays applied directly to the skin to keep tape from slipping.

Quality characteristics:
- dries quickly and adheres well

Inferior:
- irritates skin
- difficult to remove

> TIP: Essential in difficult taping situations of high humidity or where the immersion in water makes adhesiveness a problem, i.e. a swimmer returning to action.

> NOTE: May be interchanged with skin toughener spray in situations where adherence is the primary concern.

Underwrap: Pro-Wrap™; Pre-Wrap™

Applied to the taping area between "anchors", this thin foam material reduces the area of direct skin contact, protects skin from traction burns and from tape irritation. (Zinc oxide and adhesive elements in tape are frequently the cause of skin irritations or allergic reactions.)

The use of underwrap can be very helpful when taping bony areas which are particularly susceptible to skin blisters and tape cuts.

Quality characteristics:
- very fine-grained, thin foam roll that is slightly stretchy but non-adhesive. Normal width: 5 cm (2 in.)
- available in a wide range of colours as well as skintone.

Inferior:
- too thin – tears easily, tends to roll at edges producing irritating ridges if pulled over contours
- too thick – reduces efficacy of tape, not cost efficient since length of roll is significantly less as width increases

> TIP: In choosing underwrap, thinness is preferable. However, if the material is too thin, the edges tend to roll more easily, causing ridges.

> NOTE: underwrap should be used in conjunction with a spray adhesive.

Lubricating ointment: Vaseline™; Skin-Lube™

- viscous lubricating ointments used to decrease friction between tape and skin

Quality characteristics:

- maintains viscosity at body temperature
- petroleum-based

Inferior:

- thin, water-based
- will not maintain viscosity at body temperature

TIP: Care must be taken to apply only a minimal amount so that the stability and support of the entire tape job is not jeopardized.

NOTE: Lubrication is essential when taping high friction areas – e.g. the tendo-Achilles insertion – and sensitive skin areas (e.g. the front of the ankle underlaid with superficial tendons making the skin prone to blisters and/or "tape cuts".)

Heel and lace pads

- thin foam squares used in areas where there is a likelihood of friction under the taping – such as at the laces of the anterior ankle and the heel (used with a layer of skin lubricant)

Quality characteristics:

- thin but sturdy
- does not flake or break when bent
- smooth finish

Inferior:

- rough surface
- easily torn or broken

TIP: For economy, thin sheets of aerated plastic packing can be cut into 7 cm (2.75 in.) squares. Gauze squares may also be used.

Sterile gauze pads

- pads with a non-stick surface are useful for open wounds
- to cleanse abrasions and lacerations with antiseptic solution
- to protect open areas after cleaning blisters, lacerations, minor cuts and abrasions

Quality characteristics:

- firmly woven
- individually wrapped

Inferior:

- poorly packaged: unlikely to offer reliable sterility

NOTE: Be careful when opening these pads: they must be sterile when applied to a wound.

Non-sterile gauze pads

- to cleanse around abrasions and lacerations
- to apply pressure near a wound in order to arrest bleeding
- for splinting and protecting small areas such as a fractured toe

Quality characteristics:

- firmly woven

Inferior:

- flimsy weave

TIP: These pads can also be used as heel and lace pads.

Elastic bandages: Tensor™ wrap; Ace™ bandages

- one of the most versatile components of a taping kit
- a variety of different widths needed (3 in. and 6 in. are essential)
  Sizes most commonly used are:
- 15.2 cm (6 in.): support for thigh and groin strains, splint supports, holding ice packs in place, compression on soft tissue injuries, temporarily wrapping other tape jobs while adhesive "sets"
- 10 cm (4 in.): support for ankle sprains, devising a makeshift sling
- 8 cm (3 in.): small ankles; large wrists
- 5 cm (2 in.): wrist sprains; children's injuries

Quality characteristics:

- firm weave
- good elasticity: should have a wide stretch with gradually increasing resistance

TIP: There are a number of other applications where elastic bandages will prove useful. The well-appointed taping kit should have these bandages in a range of sizes and in sufficient quantity to handle diverse situations.

Taping Supplies

- good recoil: should return to within 10% of original length after use
- "clingy" surface: reduces slippage between layers and holds position on limb

Inferior:

- looser weave
- poor elasticity: stretches too easily and stops suddenly at limit of expansion
- poor recoil: tends to stay stretched after use; does not return to within 20% of original length after use
- too smooth a surface: tends to slip between layers and slides down limb

Padding: foam

- thin sheets made of dense foam
- useful when taping a bruised area: i.e. when taping a bruised tibia (shinbone) a layer of padding protects the injured area

Quality characteristics:

- "closed-cell" foam: offers good protection as it is firm in construction and waterproof

Inferior:

- thick, spongy appearance

Padding: surgical felt

- sheets of densely compressed fibres
- used as protection and support when taping a separated shoulder
- heel lifts supporting full body weight

Quality characteristics:

- firm, even texture
- soft to the touch
- equal thickness throughout sheet

Inferior:

- too loosely woven to protect adequately or to provide support when subjected to weight-bearing
- if fibres are too tightly compressed, cutting is difficult and splitting impossible
- uneven thickness over the sheet

NOTE: When effective taping requires local pressure and firm protection such as a separated shoulder, felt padding is preferable as it gives a more solid, cushioning effect than foam (A/C Shoulder separation taping see page 178). Light and tightly compacted felt is used to make heel lifts (page 124 in Chapter Six).

TIP: A thick sheet of quality felt can be split to make thinner layers.

Plastic adhesive strips: Band-Aids™

- available in a variety of widths and lengths
- packaged singly (often have non-stick sterile gauze)
- useful for simple cuts and scrapes; some brands are waterproof.
- fabric type strips also available: can be contoured to awkward surfaces - i.e. around eye

Quality characteristics:
- wrapped singly
- non-stick sterile gauze
- adhere well

Inferior:
- loosely packaged with little or no protection
- may be non-sterile
- poor adherence

Inferior fabric strips:
- poor adherence
- often stretch to the point of forming creases which may cause secondary blisters

Tape cutters
- often referred to as "sharks" because of their shape
- composed of a plastic handle encasing a replaceable razor-sharp blade
- flattened tip helps protect the skin when removing tape
- useful for cutting non-elastic tape jobs
- particularly helpful in removing ankle or wrist tapings when a scissoring action is awkward or impossible

> **TIP:** Tape cutters are essential when handling large numbers of ankle tapings and speed is critical.

Bandage scissors
- special-purpose scissors with a flattened tip that protects the underlying skin from the scissors during the tape removal process

Pen or pencil, paper (notebook preferable)
- keep an accurate record of any medical or para-medical procedure

Essential information includes:
- date of injury
- the athlete's name, team, and home phone number
- site of injury (body part)
- treatment administered and subsequent care suggested or implemented

This information is necessary for statistical records and it can also be crucial should medico-legal complications arise or if the treatment provided were to be challenged.

Surgical gloves: non-sterile; thin, disposable rubber gloves
- mandatory when attending to any bleeding or serum oozing wound. Even though an abrasion or laceration may seem insignificant, blood carries transmissible infections.
- for maximum protection, surgical gloves should be used when treating even minor injuries

Quality characteristics:
- thin yet strong
- stretch without tearing

Inferior:
- prone to tearing and puncture easily
- when ultra-thin, afford little protection in instances where the skin is broken

NOTE: When there is any doubt as to the reliability of a pair of surgical gloves, two pairs of gloves should be worn.

NOTE: Thick, clumsy gloves hinder the dexterity necessary to produce an effective taping application.

Exact change for emergency telephone call
When a major injury requires ambulance transport or supplementary medical personnel, reaction time is critical. Having the exact change for a pay-phone PLUS a list of emergency telephone numbers for the area, will facilitate summoning emergency assistance.

OPTIONAL SUPPLIES: DESCRIPTION

White zinc oxide tape: 5 cm (2 in.)
- wider tape useful in reinforcing vertical support strips (as in knee taping *see* page 138)
- edges can be folded back to significantly increase the strength of the tape

White zinc oxide tape: 1.2 cm (0.5 in.)
- narrow tape useful in taping small joints such as toes and thumbs

Adhesive remover

- dissolves adhesive and removes adhesive residue
- particularly helpful when tape has been left on longer than 24 hours

Tongue depressors: flat, wooden sticks

- useful when applying lubricants or ointments as taper's hands do not get oily

Cotton-tipped applicators: Q-Tips™

- useful in precise application of topical medication
- preferable to cotton pads or cotton balls
- use when applying skin-toughener spray to areas around the eye or near open wounds

NOTE: Spraying directly at these areas causes irritation and can be potentially dangerous.

Blister protectors: 2nd Skin™; Compeed™

- essential in the treatment of blisters
- allows the athlete to resume action while keeping the condition from deteriorating

TIP: If blister protectors are applied to vulnerable or sensitive areas prior to participation in the event, blisters are less likely to develop.

Triangular bandages: sturdy muslin squares

- useful in a wide range of situations:
  - as a sling
  - as binding material
  - as a strap for splints
  - to provide padding and/or compression

Waterproof tape

- essential in humid weather conditions or water-related events
- also effective as a waterproof covering for a tape job

Nail clippers, nail scissors

- useful when taping toes if toenails require trimming before applying tape

TAPING OBJECTIVES

The basic rationale for taping is to provide protection and support for an injured part while permitting optimal functional movement. An essential rehabilitation tool, taping enhances healing by allowing early activity within carefully controlled ranges. Taping also permits an earlier return to play or competition by protecting the area from further injury and avoiding compensatory injuries elsewhere. **Purposes** and **benefits** of correctly applied tape jobs are delineated as follows:

Purposes:
• support an injured structure
• limit harmful movements
• allow pain-free functional movement
• permit early resumption of activities

Benefits:
• circulation is enhanced through movement
• swelling is controlled
• prevents:
  a. worsening of initial injury
  b. compensatory injury to adjacent parts
  c. atrophy from non-use.
• allows:
  a. continued body conditioning and strength often lost during post-injury inactivity.
  b. maintenance of ability to react often lost due to inhibitive factors (pain, fear of re-injury)

Taping can only be truly beneficial **IF** the injury is properly assessed and the appropriate taping technique is utilized. An inappropriate tape job can place strain on associated areas, cause blisters or irritation, and, in some cases, increase the severity of the injury and cause further damage to surrounding structures.

In order to apply the tape safely and effectively, it is essential that the taper appreciate both the aims of taping and situations to avoid. In this chapter, these criteria will be outlined and discussed.

> NOTE: Taping, alone, is not a definitive treatment: for your convenience, charts hve been included in Chapter Four (Basic Pathology) and in Chapter Six – Nine (Techniques) to help put the taping in perspective relative to the entire treatment plan.

Taping Objectives

PRE-TAPING CONSIDERATIONS

By using the mnemonic **S.U.P.P.O.R.T.** to review the goals of effective taping, the taper can quickly run through a critical checklist before choosing the best technique and correlative materials for that particular injury.

S WELLING *must be controlled by adequate padding and/or compression to prevent fluids from accumulating (oedema) and to ensure the best environment for tissue regeneration and repair.*

U NDUE STRESS *to the injured region must be prevented so as to reduce the possibility of additional injury or of increasing the severity of the injury.*

P ROTECTION *of the area from further soft tissue damage (i.e. bruises, blisters, tape cuts) by using pads, lubricants and other protective materials.*

P AIN *and discomfort must be minimized by supporting the injured part, by controlling unnecessary or excessive movement, and by taking care not to cause further irritation to the injured tissues.*

O PTIMAL *healing and tissue repair can be enhanced through correctly applying tape, keeping the range of motion within safe limits, and by maintaining continuous compression.*

R EHABILITATION *of the tissues to a fully functional state (joint mobility, soft tissue flexibility, muscle strength, ligament stability and proprioception) must be considered when choosing the right taping technique adaptation for the appropriate stage of rehabilitation (subacute, functional, return to sport).*

T HERAPEUTIC CARE *in the early stages of treatment is critical for a rapid recovery. Treatment may include the application of electrical modalities (ultrasound, laser, interferential electrotherapy, muscle stimulation, etc.) to control pain and swelling and to promote rapid healing.*

POST-TAPING CONSIDERATIONS

In addition to being aware of the purposes of a particular taping application, there are conditions or situations to observe or to avoid after the taping is completed. The mnemonic **P.R.E.C.A.U.T.I.O.N.** will help recall several points important to post-taping care.

P REMATURE *participation in an activity which involves the injured part must be avoided. A major mistake many athletes make is returning to action too soon. Such activity delays healing, and often results in re-injury to the weakened structure as well as damage to compensatory areas.*

R ANGE OF MOTION *should be restricted but maintained as close as possible to the norm for the body part involved. Severe limitation of motion can result in an overextension of surrounding or compensatory structures. Permitting too free a range of motion will not adequately protect the tissues involved and will leave them prone to further injury.*

E XPERT *opinion must be obtained when any serious injury, particularly if a fracture or dislocation, is suspected. As well, there may be a paying agency's requirements or government regulations requiring a physician's assessment prior to treatment.*

C IRCULATION *in the injured area must be monitored for any sign of constriction. Pressure bandages must be checked regularly.*

A LLERGIES AND SKIN IRRITATIONS *present a very real problem – one that is frustrating for both the patient and the taper. The more serious degree of allergic reaction results in localized blistering, welts, pustules, rashes and pain. Simple irritation is generally a less severe reaction of reddened skin or small blisters.*

U NDUE DEPENDENCY ON THE TAPING *is a psychological danger which may arise when the athlete thinks he cannot perform without taping. In such cases the injured area may not return to its pre-injury performance level. Associated with this inaction, the athlete may have to spend unnecessary time in physiotherapy overcoming the results of excessive or prolonged taping.*

T ENDONS, MUSCLES AND BODY PROMINENCES *must be treated with special care and attention so as to avoid pressure build-up and friction.*

I CE *should NOT be applied to an injured part that is to be immediately subjected to taping. The temporary reduction of tissue volume due to icing will result in a taping that tightens progressively as the body part warms up. Also, an athlete may have reduced skin sensation after icing, and tissue injury can result from such sensory loss.*

O NLY *top quality supplies should be used in order to ensure a consistently high standard of tape application.*

N ERVE *conduction and local sensation may be interfered with by secondary inflammation or by the taping job itself. It is essential to evaluate the level of sensation prior to taping so that factors altering sensation can be assessed properly.*

Notes

Chapter Three

GENERAL GUIDELINES FOR TAPING

The choice of taping technique requires specific knowledge and observation skills. The following points are essential to ensure an effective, efficient taping application:

1. a thorough knowledge of anatomy
2. evaluation skills to assess – structure(s) injured
   – degree of injury
   – stage of healing
3. appropriate choice of taping technique
4. consideration of sports specific needs
5. proper preparation of the area to be taped
6. effective application of tape
7. testing the completed taping job

Deciding when to tape an injury, what techniques to apply for maximum effectiveness and how to test a completed taping job may seem a daunting task to the novice. To simplify and facilitate the process, three major stages of a taping application with useful checklists follow. These will help the taper to quickly assess all the important factors critical to each stage.

These stages are:

PRE-APPLICATION   **APPLICATION**   **POST-APPLICATION**

Using the following outline format as a guide, specific checklists for a particular sport or event may be devised with persons who are familiar with the unique requirements of the sport/event involved.

I. PRE-APPLICATION CHECKLIST

Practical: is taping going to work for this injury?
- Will tape adhere effectively to the body part?
- Is the athlete's skin damp or excessively oily?
- Are environmental factors likely to make taping impractical? (weather or sport factors – i.e. rain, cold temperatures, high humidity; diving or swimming injury)
- An athlete should not leave the treatment room with a taping job that does not stick: his/her false sense of security could lead to further injury.

Logical: is taping the correct procedure?
- Has the injury been adequately assessed? If you do not have the appropriate assessment skills, ensure that someone who does, evaluates the athlete; a) which structures are injured? b) degree of injury? c) stage of healing?
- Is there the possibility that the athlete has an unhealed fracture, an unreduced dislocation or subluxation, etc., which would require medical attention? If so, taping would not be the appropriate intervention.
- In cases of concussion, profuse bleeding, abrasion, laceration, etc, **FIRST AID** is the treatment of choice – not taping.

Materials: what is needed?
A quick review of the type and quantity of taping materials needed for the specific injury at hand will facilitate a swift, organized taping job. Having the materials ready and within reach will maximize efficiency.

Assessment: what is injured or at risk?
The ability to assess which body structures are injured (or at risk, either directly or indirectly), and to what degree, is essential in selecting the right taping application. A thorough knowledge of anatomy coupled with an understanding of the demands and requirements of specific sports are also essential elements in determining the appropriate taping technique. Application of this knowledge will become second nature through experience.

> NOTE: Should an athlete continue to participate in his/her sport with an improperly diagnosed injury, the result could be serious tissue damage and a complicated recovery process.

> TIP: A general first aid course is highly recommended for anyone involved in the treatment of sports-related injuries.

> TIP: Practising on simulated injuries helps improve decision making and taping skills.

*The following general points should be considered **before** taping an injury:*

Joint range and muscle flexibility: what is the athlete's norm?

Although this range differs from athlete to athlete, testing and examination of the corresponding uninjured joint and muscle area should be helpful in delineating these factors. This procedure will also ensure that the taping will not excessively limit the range of motion of the injured area.

Problem areas: superficial skin damage in creases or bony areas.

Soft skin (in elbow or knee creases) and areas where tape pulls around bony points (the back of the heel in ankle taping), are often the sites of superficial skin damage.

Constant pressure form a poor tape job can cause painful pressure points (such as the base of the fifth metatarsal bone when an ankle is taped too tightly).

Arteries or bones that are anatomically superficial, (close to the skin surface) require extra care to avoid skin damage.

Trouble spots for each injury area should be reviewed before taping is attempted.

Sport-specific items: meeting movement demands of the athlete.

What is the range of motion required for the injured athlete's sport? Each position on the team demands different types of movement from any one joint. For example, for a lateral ankle sprain, when taping a basketball player, the taping need is near-maximum plantarflexion (for jumping); in taping an ice hockey player, the requirement shifts to near-maximum dorsiflexion. In both cases the taping purpose is to prevent abnormal lateral mobility, yet the taping procedures must be different in order to accommodate the demands of a sport-specific range of motion.

The starting position of the injured part in preparation for taping.

The best position is one in which the injured structure is unstressed (or neutral), and well-supported, (not stretched). Check that the athlete is sufficiently comfortable to maintain the required position throughout the taping procedure. The taper should also be able to work from an efficient, comfortable, biomechanically sound position.

II. APPLICATION CHECKLIST

Preparation of the injured area.

Skin Condition:

Dirty: clean gently with a liquid antiseptic soap or antiseptic-soaked gauze. Pat dry. If skin is lacerated or abrased, apply a light layer of antibiotic ointment locally and cover with protective gauze.

Wet: dry gently with gauze. Use adhesive spray.

Oily: wipe with rubbing alcohol-soaked gauze. Apply adhesive spray to ensure tape adhesion.

Hairy: shave area to be taped. Apply antiseptic lotion. Swab dry with gauze. Use a skin toughener if skin is not irritated.

Irritated: apply a small amount of antibiotic ointment.
Apply lubricant sparingly and use protective padding over the area.

> TIP: In all taping procedures, protective layers with a lubricant should be used in areas particularly susceptible to irritation from taping, such as the back of the heel, ankles, hamstring tendons, and knee tapings.

Choosing the correct tape for a specific taping job.

As stated in Chapter Two, choosing the right type of tape depends on the actual structure(s) involved and whether the taping job involves padding, support, restraint or compression.

In general, **ELASTIC** tape is used for **contractile** tissue injuries (i.e. muscles, tendons). Elastic tape is preferable in these instances because it gives stretch with support and a graduated resistance, yet limits full stretch of the muscle or tendon.

Because muscles must be allowed a certain amount of normal expansion during activity, **elastic** tape should be used as **anchors** when encircling muscle bulk is required.

Elastic tape should also be used for specific **compression** taping requiring localised pressure. **NON-ELASTIC** tape is used to support injuries of **non-contractile** structures (i.e. ligaments). Non-elastic tape reinforces the joints in the same way the ligaments would, thereby increasing joint stability.

Taping application.

The person applying tape to an injury must modify the application to suit the circumstances specific to each situation. Education and experience will enable the taper to develop variations on the basic techniques offered in this guide. Several ankle taping variations are illustrated in Chapter Six.

As long as the tape application is fulfilling the taping goal of supporting or protecting the targeted area without putting other structures at risk, a procedural variation can be used.

Taping techniques

The two main techniques used in applying tape are commonly referred to as **strip** taping and **smooth roll**.

"Strip" taping employs one short strip of tape at a time, in very specific directions and with highly controlled tension.

This technique is often used in basic preventative taping as demonstrated in Chapter Six.

"Smooth roll" refers to use of a single, continuous, uninterrupted winding of a piece of tape.

	Advantages	Disadvantages
Strip	• Accurate tension • Tape applied only where needed.	• Requires time and practice
Smooth roll	• Quick to apply • Useful when taping an entire team	• Difficult to control tension • Tendency to use too much tape

NOTE: The "strip" technique is demonstrated in this guide as the authors believe this technique to be more effective as it provides very specific localised support for the injured structures.

Quality control: While the taping is in progress, monitor these points:

- is effective compression being maintained without loss of circulation?
- is the tape adhering properly?
- is the injured structure being properly supported by the technique chosen?
- are the supporting strips adequately tight?

III. POST-APPLICATION CHECKLIST

Monitoring the results: is the taping effective?
Follow these steps only when the tape job has been completed:
- gently manually stress the joint movement to check for adequate limitation at the extremes of range of motion and in the direction of the injury.
- check for stability of the joint and of the taping strips. The athlete should experience no pain during these tests.
- further testing of the finished taping procedure involves functional tests in sport-specific movements as well as action and/or ranges of motion.

Functional testing: can the athlete safely engage in his sport?
Before the athlete can return to the playing field, it is necessary to thoroughly evaluate the taping relative to performance of sport-specific skills and movements.
These tests, performed in order of increasing difficulty and stress to the joints, should be assessed by the athlete's medical support personnel.

Example:
Sport: soccer
Injured area: ankle
Testing progression:
- simple walking to jogging
- then running in a straight line
- running in a loose "S" line
- running in a tight "S" line
- running in a figure "8"
- cutting side to side at a jog (zig-zag)
- cutting side to side at a run
- running backwards
- finally, jumping.

NOTE: At this point in testing, any ineffective taping should either be adjusted to correct the problem that is causing the pain or loss of agility or be completely reapplied. The injury should be reassessed for appropriateness of taping.

The last activity will test the athlete's ability to perform full weightbearing on the ankle from a height - a position which places the ankle at its highest risk of re-injury.
If at any juncture in these tests the athlete experiences pain or loss of agility, the evaluation should be stopped before the athlete suffers further injury or re-injury.

General Guidelines for Taping

The key factors in determining whether or not the athlete can return to participation are:
- monitoring ability and speed in sport-specific skills
- pain-free functional testing.

Tape removal:
When a tape application is no longer required, removal of the tape job must be done carefully. The "tear-it-off-quick-before-you-know-it!" temptation should be avoided. This method causes skin damage jeopardizing subsequent or follow-up taping applications.

For speed and ease of tape removal, bandage scissors or special tape cutters (the "sharks" mentioned previously) should be used so as to avoid damage to skin and other sensitive structures in the area.

The preferred method is to first cut the tape: Using the blunt tip of the scissors, ease the skin away from the adhering tape, forming a "tunnel" to facilitate cutting.

The tape is then peeled off slowly and *gently*, while pressing down on the exposed skin and pulling the tape back on itself, parallel - *not* perpendicular - to the surface of the skin.

Are there any signs of skin irritation or breakdown?
The skin must be inspected closely for signs of irritation, blisters, or other types of allergic reaction.

> TIP: A small amount of lubricant on the tip of the cutting instrument will help it to glide underneath the tape.

Chapter Four ....

BASIC PATHOLOGY

The majority of injuries incurred during participation in sports activities are sprains, strains and contusions involving the musculo-skeletal system. The taping techniques demonstrated in this guide are particularly helpful for these conditions. Although some form of splinting and protection is also necessary for fractures, dislocations, nerve injuries, lacerations, abrasions and blisters, these conditions are beyond the intended scope of this guide.

The structures most often requiring taping are joints, ligaments, muscles, tendons, and associated bony parts. The following brief description of these structures with specific taping considerations will help the beginner and serve as a review for the more advanced taper.

Joints:

these are structures formed where two or more bones meet and move one on another. The lateral movements of joints are controlled by ligaments. Friction is minimized by the smooth cartilage over the articulated surface of the bone and by the synovial joint capsule.

Because of the complex interaction of muscles and tendons involved in joint movement, an injury to any link in the functional chain unbalances the entire structure. This imbalance causes pain and varying degrees of joint dysfunction. Therefore, in taping joints, the primary concern is to support and protect the injured structure. Reestablishing the joint's delicate balance while optimizing mobility without shifting function and/or reliance to compensatory structures is also very important.

When a joint has been taped, the athlete must go through sport-specific movements to determine that joint balance has been restored and to evaluate compensatory stress. The athlete should be able to perform all required motions without experiencing pain.

Ligaments:

these are non-elastic connective tissue structures that stabilize joints and reinforce joint capsules. When ligaments are stretched, torn, or bruised, the resulting sprain requires careful taping in order to reestablish structural support and functional movement to the joint while preventing or reducing the threat of further stretch to the ligament. Generally, a **non-elastic** taping application that appropriately restricts unwanted movement of the joint involved will allow the ligament to recover without further stress or trauma.

Muscle/tendon units:

these are elastic contractile structures that produce movement of the musclo-skeletal system.

An elastic taping application provides resilient support while limiting full stretch of the injured structure. Elastic tape also allows normal changes in structure girth while maintaining compression, thus vital circulation to the limb involved is not jeopardized.

Bony prominences:

these are superficial bony areas with little overlying soft tissue.

These areas require special care when taping as these prominent points easily develop skin blisters and abrasions under tape because they lack subcutaneous protection.

If tape strips are applied too tightly over these bony areas, the compression can result in compromised circulation, neural compression, or acute pain leading to impaired performance.

USEFUL MNEMONIC

As discussed in Chapter Three, before beginning any taping procedure it is important to properly assess the injured region in order to determine the most appropriate treatment and taping application. The following material is presented in a format designed to facilitate a simple, quick method of assessment of the degree of injury in three areas: **sprains, strains, contusions.** Similar charts for specific injuries are included in Chapters Six–Nine following each of the taping techniques illustrated. Should there be any uncertainty concerning the severity of any particular condition, further medical evaluation and investigation must be sought. It is the responsibility of the taper to recommend such further medical care.

Using the mnemonic T.E.S.T.S. in assessing injured structures:
The authors have devised a simple order of assessment steps with an mnemonic to assist the reader. **T.E.S.T.S.** stands for:

T ERMINOLOGY: proper names, synonyms and other pertinent information for identifying an injury or condition.

E TIOLOGY: relative mechanisms, causitive factors, prevalence.

S YMPTOMS: • subjective complaints of the injured athlete including a description of the injury.
• objective physical findings which can be measured by the taper.

T REATMENT: includes early and later phases of first aid, physiotherapy, taping; medical follow-up when necessary.

S EQUELAE: possible complications that can result if the original condition is left untreated, or is poorly treated, or if adequate expert medical follow-up is not pursued.

The following three charts are intended to clarify the classification and degree of an injury. They outline the various aspects of treatment and put the taping procedures in perspective relative to the total treatment plan. Taping, alone, is not a definitive treatment, but rather a protection and a means to facilitate a safe, speedy recovery.

> **NOTE:** Using the mnemonic R.I.C.E.S., one can easily remember the basic treatment elements for acute soft tissue injuries: Rest, Ice, Compression, Elevation, Support.

SPRAINS: INJURY TO A LIGAMENTOUS STRUCTURE

	FIRST DEGREE	SECOND DEGREE	THIRD DEGREE
Terminology	FIRST DEGREE: fibre damage with little or no elongation	SECOND DEGREE: overstretch with partial tearing causing moderate to major elongation	THIRD DEGREE: complete rupture
Etiology	mild direct or indirect stress to a ligament	moderate stress to a ligament	severe stress to one or more ligaments
Symptoms	• some pain at rest possible • some pain on active movement (in direction of trauma) • some pain on resisted movement (in direction of trauma) • some pain on passive movement (in direction of trauma) • pain on stress testing of injured ligament • some swelling • some discolouration • no instability • minimal loss of function	• localized and/or diffuse pain even at rest • pain on active movement (direction of injury) • pain on resisted movement (multi-directional) • pain on passive stretch (in direction of injury) • exquisite tenderness at site of injury • significant swelling • discolouration not always present immediately • marked pain on stressing ligament • demonstrable laxity on stress testing • slight to significant loss of structural integrity • mild to moderate loss of dynamic function	• often less painful than 2nd degree due to complete rupture of ligament • marked swelling • discolouration common • significantly abnormal movement on stress testing • major loss of structural integrity • major loss of structural function
Treatment: early later	• R.I.C.E.S. first 48 hours • taped support • therapeutic modalities • range of motion continued physiotherapy including: • taped support: 3–10 days until pain-free • activity permitted (with taping) if no pain • strengthening exercises (isometric at first) • proprioception	• R.I.C.E.S. for first 48 hours • taped support allowing for possible swelling • non-weightbearing first 48 hours. • therapeutic modalities• continued physiotherapy including: • mobilization if stiff • transverse friction massage if local swelling and stiffness • isometric strengthening • modified activity for 2–3 weeks followed by closely monitored return to activity if pain-free with taped support • continue taping 4–6 weeks • proprioceptive re-eduction crucial to avoiding re-injury • total rehabilitation program to restore range of motion, flexibility, strength, balance coordination and proprioception	• R.I.C.E.S. for first 48 hours • taped support • often requires surgery, bracing or casting with fibreglass or plaster physiotherapy including: • therapeutic modalities • mobilizations if stiff (post-immobilization) • flexibility • strengthening (isometric at first with the joint in neutral position) • modified exercise program to maintain fitness level throughout treatment • gradual pain-free reintegration program with taped support • continued taped support for at least 4 months • ligaments require up to one year to regain full tensile strength • total rehabilitation program as for 2nd degree with emphasis on proprioception: 2–3 months
Sequelae	• chronic pain at site of injury • re-injury • weakness • stiffness	• chronically unstable or 'lax' joint • chronic pain • re-injury • reduced proprioception • weakness • arthritic changes	• adhesions • prolonged disability • instability if ligament heals in a lengthened position • high probability of re-injury if rehabilitation is incomplete • weakness • reduced proprioception and reaction ability • arthritic complications

R.I.C.E.S. : Rest, Ice, Compress, Elevate, Support

SPRAINS: INJURY TO ANY PART OF A MUCULOTENDINOUS UNIT

Terminology	FIRST DEGREE: fibre damage with little or no elongation	SECOND DEGREE: partial tearing of fibres causing moderate to major elongation	THIRD DEGREE: complete rupture
Etiology	• mild to moderate stress against muscle contraction • mild to moderate overstretching • unaccustomed activity • lack of warmup	• moderate to severe stress against muscle contraction • moderate to severe overstretching • unaccustomed resisted, repetitive activity	• severe stress against a muscle contraction • explosive muscle contraction causing spontaneous contraction of the antagonist muscle during vigorous physical activity ('hamstring' strains in sprinters; calf strains in tennis players) • severe overstretching • improper warmup and/or pre-activity stretching • weakened tendons from repeated cortisone injections
Symptoms	• mild local or diffuse pain • some swelling • some discolouration possible • pain on active contraction • increased pain on resistance • increased pain on passive stretch • pain on local palpation • minimal loss of function	• moderate to major pain, localized and/or diffuse • moderate swelling • discolouration not apparent if intramuscular • moderate to major pain on active contraction • moderate to severe pain on resistance • moderate to major weakness • moderate to severe pain on passive stretch • spasm • pain localized on palpation • moderate to major loss of function	• often minimal pain due to complete rupture • marked swelling • discolouration varies with injury site • no significant pain on active contraction • zero strength on selective testing • 'bunching' of muscle can cause bump & hollow deformity • total loss of function
Treatment: early	• R.I.C.E.S. for first 48 hours • taping to prevent full stretch and to give elastic support to musculo-tendinous unit (compression taping over muscle belly if injury site is in muscle bulk). See compression taping for calf Chapter 6 or quads Chapter 7 • weight-bearing only if pain-free • therapeutic modalities	• R.I.C.E.S. for first 48 hours • taping as for 1st degree; compression taping over muscle belly if injury site is in muscle belly • non-weightbearing during first 48 hours. or until pain-free • therapeutic modalities • active contraction of antagonist (opposite) muscle to induce relaxation, flexibility and eliminate spasm	• R.I.C.E.S. for first 48 hours • taping support to shorten structure: 3 weeks immobilization • surgery or casting in a shortened position often recommended
later	continued physiotherapy including: • flexibility exercises • progressive strengthening • controlled activity with taped support • continue taping for 1–3 weeks • transverse friction massage for adhesions • rapid return to full pain-free activity • total rehabilitation program for strength, flexibility and proprioception	continued physiotherapy including: • flexibility exercises • strengthening exercises • transverse friction massage for adhesions • modified exercise program to maintain fitness • gradual pain-free reintegration to full activity with taped support • continue taping for 3–6 weeks	physiotherapy including: • therapeutic modalities • modified exercise program to maintain fitness • flexibility exercises • strengthening exercises: begin with isometric progressing to eccentric and concentric • gradual reintegration to full pain-free physical activity with taped support; continue taping for 8–12 weeks • total rehabilitation program for flexibility, strength and proprioception
Sequelae	• chronic pain • scarring • inflexibility • weakness • re-injury	• chronic pain • scarring • inflexibility • weakness and inhibition • prone to tendinitis • re-injury possibly causing complete rupture	• scarring • inflexibility • weakness • significant loss of function should healing take place while muscle is in a lengthened position • reduced reaction ability

R.I.C.E.S. : Rest, Ice, Compress, Elevate, Support

Basic Pathology

CONTUSIONS: CRUSHING INJURY TO SOFT TISSUE (CAN BE INTRA-MUSCULAR OR INTER-MUSCULAR)

Terminology	FIRST DEGREE: minor soft tissue crushing	SECOND DEGREE: moderately strong direct blow causing moderate trauma and bruising	THIRD DEGREE: major soft tissue damage
Etiology	mild direct or indirect blow causing bruising	moderately strong direct blow causing moderate trauma and bruising	hard direct blow – usually to the muscle belly, causing severe trauma and major bleeding
Symptoms	• localized pain • minimal swelling • some discolouration possible if intra-muscular • range of motion usually not significantly affected • some pain on active movement • some pain on resistance • some pain on passive stretch • tender on palpation • athletic ability generally not restricted	• significant diffuse and localized pain • noticeable swelling • discolouration if intermuscular • restricted range of motion due to pain and swelling • moderate to major pain on active contraction • major pain on resistance • weakness • major pain on passive stretch • tender on palpation • moderate loss of function	• severe pain • extensive swelling • discolouration if inter-muscular • very limited range of motion • pain on active contraction • marked spasm • often a palpable deformity at injury site or a palpable fluid mass if intra-muscular
Treatment: early	• R.I.C.E.S. for first 48 hours • immediate taped support: See compression taping for calf Chapter 6 or quads Chapter 7 • active contraction of opposing muscles to restore full flexibility	• R.I.C.E.S. for first 48 hours • immediate taped support: See compression taping for calf Chapter 6 or quads Chapter 7 • therapeutic modalities	• R.I.C.E.S. for first 48 hours • immediate taped support. See compression taping for calf Chapter 6 or quads Chapter 7 • complete rest • leg injuries require crutches • therapeutic modalities • active isometric contraction of antagonist muscles peripheral to injury site to induce pain-free stretching
later	continued physiotherapy including: • flexibility • strengthening • transverse friction massage for adhesions • controlled activity with compressive support • continue taping 3–10 days until pain-free	continued physiotherapy including: • cautious progression of pain-free strengthening exercises • active contraction of antagonist muscles to induce pain-free stretching of the injured muscle	continued physiotherapy including: • flexibility exercises • no massage during first 3 weeks • transverse friction massages for adhesions only in later remodelling stage (4 weeks) • cautious progression of pain-free strengthening exercises with taped support • controlled, gradual pain-free progression of activity with taped support • continued compression for at least 4–8 weeks
Sequelae	• cramping • scarring • loss of flexibility • re-injury	• traumatic myositis ossificans (bone formation within the muscle) often caused by aggressive, premature massage, heat and/or stretching • scarring • inflexibility • permanent weakness • deformity	• traumatic myositis ossificans (bone formation within the muscle) often caused by aggressive, premature massage, heat, and/or stretching • scarring • inflexibility • permanent weakness • deformity • risk of spontaneous rupture

R.I.C.E.S. : Rest, Ice, Compress, Elevate, Support

Chapter Five

KEY TAPING TECHNIQUES

Most taping applications are variations on basic key taping strategies. The differences in taping techniques lie in the manner and direction of the application of each strip of tape and the type of taping material utilized. Each particular taping strategy has to meet the multiple requirements of a particular sport, the type of joint and related structure(s) to be taped, as well as the type and severity of the injury the athlete has sustained.

This short chapter will familiarize the reader with the most common elements of our taping strategies including the functional descriptive names of individual strips of tape, their purpose, and method of application.

The strips illustrated include:

- anchors
- stirrups
- vertical
- "butterfly" or check-rein
- locks
- figure-8
- compression
- closing-up

TAPE RIPPING:

Before attempting these strips, it is worthwhile to learn how to rip tape efficiently. **Tape ripping** *is an acquired skill and not as easy as it sounds! The steps shown in the two photographs on the left will be useful in learning this practical skill.*

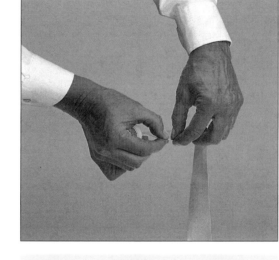

1. *Pinch the tape edge firmly with the thumbnails adjacent (back to back and perpendicular to the tape).*

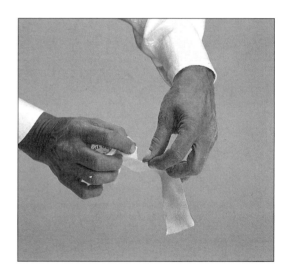

2. *Make a sudden jerking movement by sharply shearing your hands in opposite directions while maintaining tension on the tape edge.*

PREPARATION OF PRACTICE STRIPS:

To acquire taping skills, **practice strips** should be prepared. Because the precise applications of Figure 8 and locking strips are tricky to learn, it is advisable to apply numerous practice strips to perfect the technique. This practice strip can be stuck to the limb as though it were a regular strip and the various complicated techniques can be practiced without wasting tape. By experimenting with the "take-off" angle and the degree on lateral shearing, the taper can learn to accommodate for the varieties of ankle shapes and thickness. It is important to be able to control the direction of the strip and thus adapt the final supporting result.

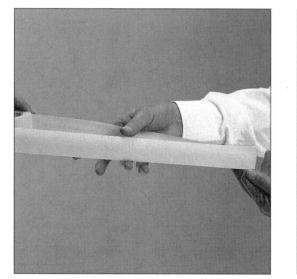

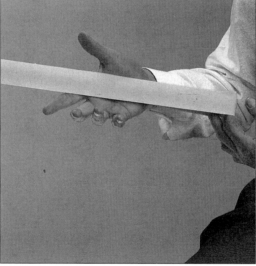

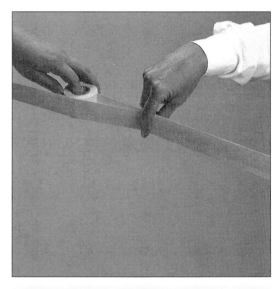

1. *Unroll 1 meter (3 ft) of tape and have a helper hold it at one end.*
2. *Hold the tape with two fingers (slightly separated) with your left hand while your helper unrolls another 1 meter (3 ft) of tape.*

3. *Guide these two pieces of parallel tape (sticky side in) so that they meet without overlapping.*
4. *While maintaining tension on the tape gently press one strip against the other throughout the length of the tape while controlling the tension to avoid wrinkles and overlapping.*

5. *Remove your fingers from the loop end of the tape and stick the sides together.*
6. *Finish sticking the other end of the tape and remove from the roll leaving one side 15 cm (6 in.) longer than the original piece with one sticky side.*

COMMONLY USED TAPE STRIPS:

ANCHORS

Description: the first tape strips applied for each tape job. They may be either non-elastic or elastic tape, depending on expansion requirements of the underlying structures.

Purpose: to form a stable base for subsequent supporting strips of tape.

Method: place these tape strips around the circumference of the limb to be supported, both above and below the injury. They must be placed directly on the skin, and must follow anatomical contours for optimal adherence.

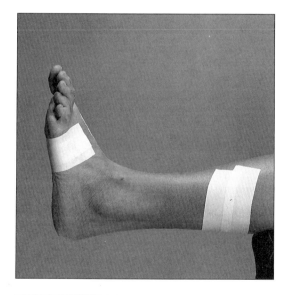

non-elastic tape anchors

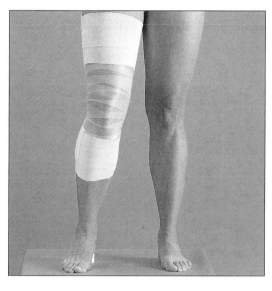

elastic tape anchors

STIRRUPS:

Description: a U-shaped loop of non-elastic tape.

Purpose: to directly support an injured ligament.

Method: place the tape so that a lateral and a medial component lend stability. Pull the tape tighter on the injured side.

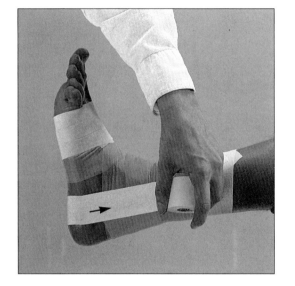
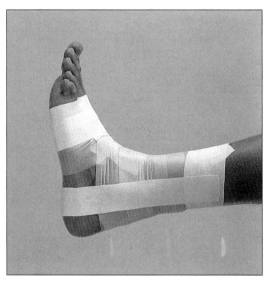

VERTICAL STRIPS:

Description: non-elastic tape strips applied under tension from one anchor to the other.

Purpose: to limit lateral mobility by drawing the distal segment of the injured structure towards the proximal.

Method: affix one end of vertical strip to distal anchor and apply tension over the injured structure while affixing tape to the proximal anchor.

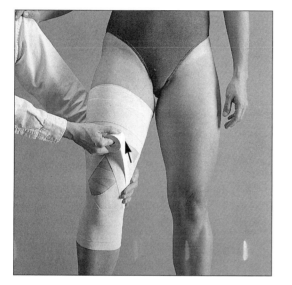
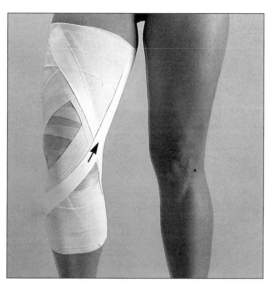

"BUTTERFLY" OR CHECK-REIN:

Description: a combination of three or more vertical strips applied at angles of 10° to 45° to each other, placed at the axis of rotation of the joint to be taped. These strips can be of either non-elastic or elastic tape depending on the injured structure and the goals of the taping.

Purpose: to restrict movement in more than a simple uniplanar direction, as so often found in normal motion. This "butterfly" or "check-rein" can resist stresses with inherent torsion components as well as those that are purely unidirectional.

Method: Steps in applying "butterfly" strips:

NOTE: Proper positioning of the injured limb is crucial to effective application.

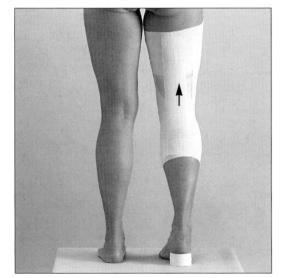

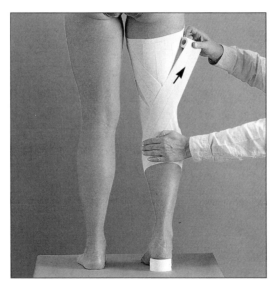

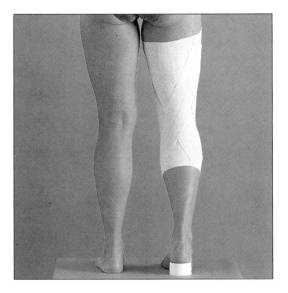

first strip: *in a truly vertical position from the distal anchor to the proximal anchor.*

second strip: *in a slightly rotated fashion in one direction*

third strip: *in a slightly rotated position opposite to the second strip.*

final step: *reanchor these strips*

NOTE: The axis of the three strips lies directly on the joint line.

LOCKS:

Description: a **non-elastic** tape strip attached firmly to the underlying anchors reinforcing support.

Purpose: to reinforce joint stability yet allow protected, functional movements.

Method: strong tension is applied at key points in the application of the locking strip which reinforces the injured structure and stabilizes the joint.

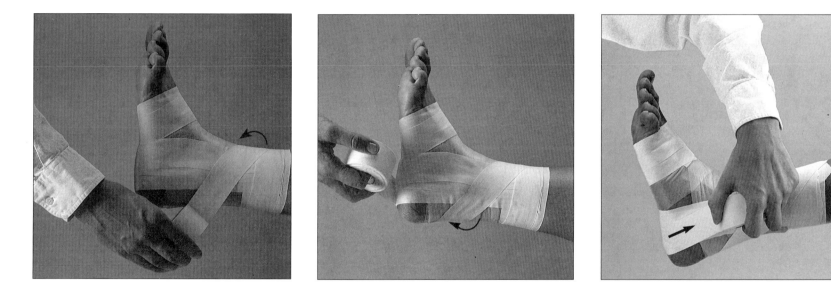

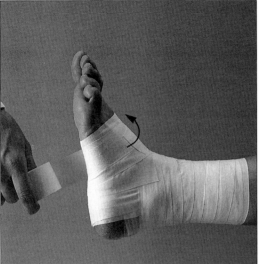

FIGURE-8

Description: a strip of non-elastic tape forming a figure-8; usually applied as one of the last strips in an ankle or thumb taping.

Purpose: to give added stability; to cover any remaining open areas and/or tape ends; to close the tape application neatly.

Method: apply the tape by encircling one segment of the limb in one direction before crossing over to encircle the adjacent segment in the opposite direction, thus forming a "figure 8".

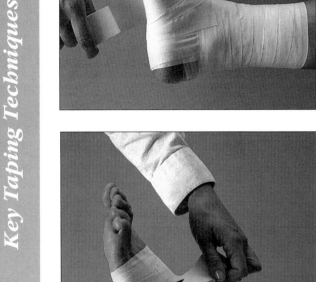

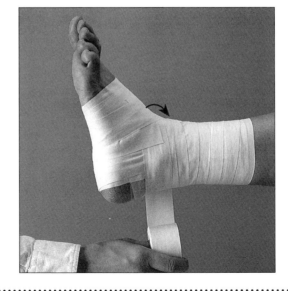

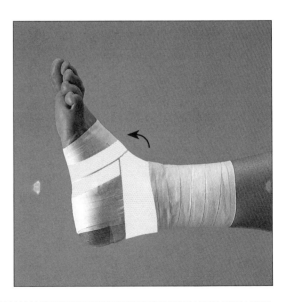

COMPRESSION STRIPS:

Description: elastic adhesive tape strips applied with localized compression over a muscle injury.

Purpose:
- to provide strong compressive forces localized to the injured area
- to minimise subsequent swelling
- to prevent further injury without compromising circulation.
- to permit activity

Method:
- apply one layer of elastic adhesive tape directly to the skin with minimal tension to form a base.
- apply pressure strips by holding the tape fully stretched while pressing firmly directly over the injury. Maintain the pressure while **gradually** releasing it behind the limb before overlapping the ends **without tension** to avoid a tourniquet effect. Repeat the compression strips with each overlapping the previous one by half until the entire injured area - distal (lower) to proximal (upper) -is covered.

NOTE: It is essential that the tension is released completely posteriorly before closing each tape strip.

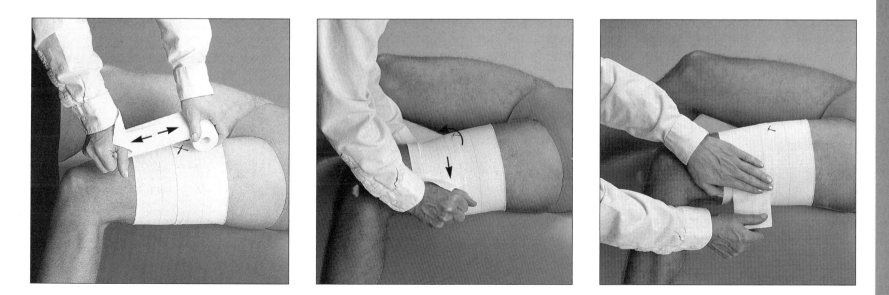

CLOSING-UP STRIPS:

Description: lightly placed strips of either elastic or non-elastic tape, which cover any remaining open areas or tape ends, neatly finishing the taping job.

Purpose:
- to reduce the risk of skin blisters by covering all open areas.
- to make the tape job less likely to unravel during athletic activity.
- to give a neat appearance to the finished taping.

Method: apply the strips of tape around the circumference of the limb, with a one-third to one-half width of overlap, starting proximally (upper end) and moving distally (lower end)

NOTE: By applying these strips from proximal to distal, the tape edges will not be pulled or rolled back when the athlete rapidly dresses for sport after taping.

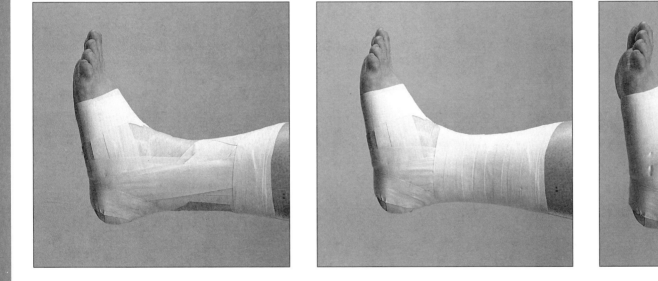
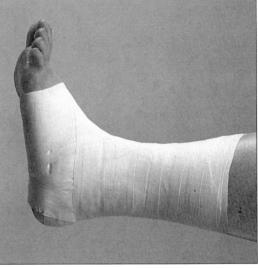

Chapter Six

FOOT AND ANKLE

The procedures for taping the majority of sports injuries are illustrated in this and the following chapters. The intent of these procedures is to provide protection while allowing functional movement thus preventing further damage to the injured structure or adjacent areas. Inherent in each approach, and essential to accurate assessment of every injury, are medical diagnosis, treatment and appropriate follow-up.

T.E.S.T.S. charts in this section put each taping technique into perspective relative to total injury management. They include key points under the headings of **T**erminology, **E**tiology, **S**ymptoms, **T**reatment and **S**equelae. These charts are meant as helpful guides and are not to be considered as in-depth analyses with all possible complications.

A thorough understanding of the techniques illustrated in these chapters combined with experience in handling a wide range of injuries, will enable the taper to adapt and apply effective taping techniques to the many unusual and/or challenging situations which inevitably arise.

ANATOMICAL AREA: FOOT AND ANKLE

FOOT AND ANKLE TAPING TECHNIQUES

The articulations of the foot and ankle are numerous and complex. The joints of the foot and curvature of the arches of the foot permit adaptation to irregular terrain. These joints offer suppleness and shock absorption through elasticity. This varied bony architecture and mobility predisposes to different types of injuries. Taped support can alleviate many stresses related to these conditions.

The **talo-crural** (the true ankle) joint is mainly responsible for dorsiflexion and plantar flexion while the **sub-talar joint** allows more lateral mobility – inversion and eversion – (sideways deviation) permitting the foot to adapt to all angles of incline or slope. This relatively mobile **ankle joint** complex is dependent on numerous ligaments for its stability, and on tendons for its dynamic support. Forces through this relatively fragile joint make it vulnerable to stresses. The ankle is most easily injured during weightbearing activities which require quick changes of direction.

A variety of taping techniques are highly effective in supporting both ligamentous and musculo-tendinous conditions related to the ankle joint. With the application of proper taping techniques, the athlete can rapidly resume normal competitive activity and/or intense training.

In this and the following chapters, details on the following items will prove useful:

- specific purpose of each taping technique
- conditions appropriate for specific applications
- a list of materials
- special notes
- positioning for taping procedure
- illustrated procedure
- highly informative sidebar tips
- a sample condition (injury) in a T.E.S.T.S. chart form

Section Two

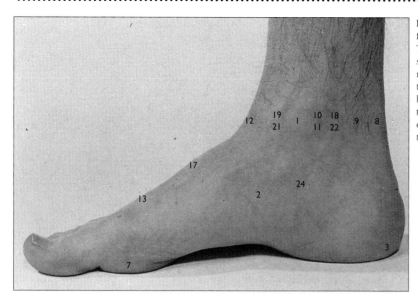

Right ankle and foot, from the medial side.
The most prominent surface features are the medial malleolus, the tendo calcaneus at the back and the tendons of tibialis anterior and extensor hallucis longus at the front.

Right ankle and foot, from the lateral side. The most prominent surface features are the lateral malleolus the tendo calcaneus at the back and the tendon of tibialis anterior at the front.

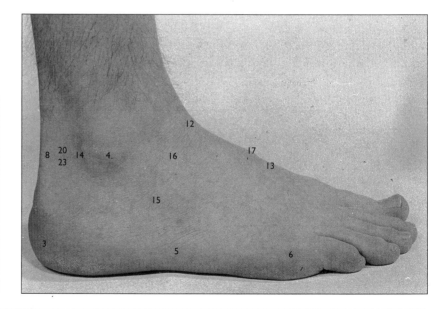

SURFACE ANATOMY	
BONES	13 EXTENSOR HALLUCIS LONGUS
1 MEDIAL MALLEOUS	14 PERONEUS LONGUS AND BREVIS
2 TUBEROSITY OF NAVICUALR	15 EXTENSOR DIGITORUM BREVIS
3 TUBEROSITY OF CALCANEUS	16 EXTENSOR DIGITORUM LONGUS
4 LATERAL MALLEOLUS	**ARTERIES**
5 TUBEROSITY OF BASE OF 5th METATARSAL	17 DORSALIS PEDIS
6 HEAD OF 5th METATARSAL	18 POSTERIOR TIBIAL
7 SESAMOID BONE	**VEINS**
TENDONS	19 GREAT SAPHENEOUS
8 TENDO CALCANEUS (ACHILLES)	20 SMALL SAPHENEOUS
9 FLEXOR HALLUCIS LONGUS	**NERVES**
10 FLEXOR DIGITORUM LONGUS	21 GREAT SAPHENEOUS
11 TIBIALIS POSTERIOR	22 POSTERIOR TIBIAL
12 TIBIALIS ANTERIOR	23 SURAL
	LIGAMENTS
	24 SUSTENTACULUM TALI

Foot and Ankle

DEEP DISSECTION

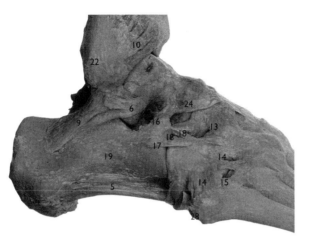

LATERAL VIEW

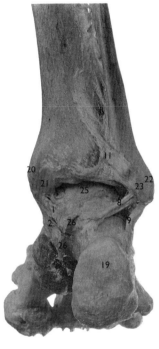

POSTERIOR VIEW

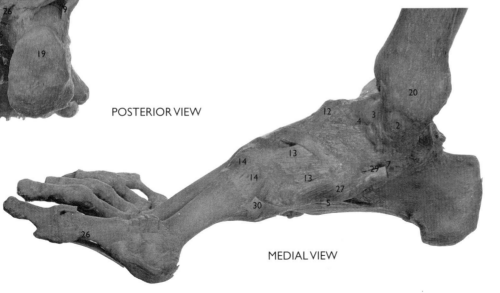

MEDIAL VIEW

LIGAMENTS
DELTOID LIGAMENT:
  1 POSTERIOR TIBIOTALAR PART
  2 TIBIOCALCANEAN PART
  3 ANTERIOR TIBIOTALAR PART
  4 TIBIONAVICULAR PART
5 LONG PLANTAR LIGAMENT
6 ANTERIOR TALOFIBULAR
7 SUSTENTACULUM TALI
8 POSTERIOR TALO FIBULAR
9 CALCANEO FIBULAR
10 ANTERIOR INFERIOR TIBIOFIBULAR
11 POSTERIOR INFERIOR TIBIOFIBULAR
12 TALO NAVICULAR
13 DORSAL CUNEONAVICULAR
14 DORSAL TARSO-METATARSAL
15 DORSAL METATARSAL
16 CERVICAL
17 DORSAL CALCANEO CUBOID
18 BIFURCATE (CALCANEO CUBOID AND CALCANEO NAVICULAR PARTS)

BONES
19 CALCANEUS
20 MEDIAL MALLEOLUS OF THE TIBIA
21 GROOVE FOR TIBIALIS POSTERIOR TENDON
22 LATERAL MALLEOLUS OF TIBIA
23 GROOVE FOR PERONEUS BREVIS TENDON
24 HEAD OF TALUS
25 TROCHLEAR SURFACE OF TALUS
26 GROOVE FOR FLEXOR HALLUCIS LONGUS TENDON
27 TUBEROSITY OF NAVICULAR
28 TUBEROSITY OF BASE OF 5TH METATARSAL

TENDONS
29 TIBIALIS POSTERIOR
30 TIBIALIS ANTERIOR
31 PERONEUS LONGUS
32 FLEXOR HALLUCIS LONGUS

TAPING FOR TOE SPRAIN

Purpose:
- support of first metatarsophalangeal (MTP) joint
- allows moderate flexion and some extension
- limits end range of flexion, extension, adduction

Indications for use:
- sprains of first metatarsophalangeal (MTP) joint
- for a medial collateral ligament sprain: abduct the toe and reinforce the medial restraining tape strips.
- for a plantar ligament sprain (hyperextension injury): reinforce the **X** on the plantar surface to limit extension.
- for a lateral collateral ligament sprain: reinforce with buddy taping to the first toe. (**For an example of buddy taping used with fingers – *see* page 218**)
- for a dorsal capsular sprain (hyperflexion): reinforce the **X** on the dorsal suface to limit flexion.
- hyperflexion of first MTP joint: "turf toe"
- contusion of first MTP joint: "jammed toe", "stubbed toe"
- painful bunions

MATERIALS:

razor
skin toughener spray
2 cm (3/4 in.) white tape (or split 3.8 cm (1.5 in.)tape)

> **NOTES**
> - The base of the fifth metatarsal bone is a sensitive, vulnerable area prone to pressure pain and blisters if tape is tight.
> - To avoid constriction, minimal tension must be used when wrapping circumference anchors.
> - Application of lubricant to adjacent toes and/or the inside of the toe box of the shoe will prevent chafing.
> - Trimming toenails will lessen the risk of irritation.
> - Careful application of a minimum amount of tape is particularly important when taping for sports that require tight-fitting shoes or boots.

For additional details regarding an injury example see TESTS chart page 56.

Positioning:

Sitting on treatment table with injured foot slightly overhanging the end of the table.

Procedure:

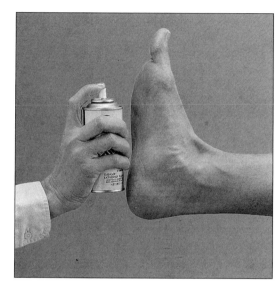

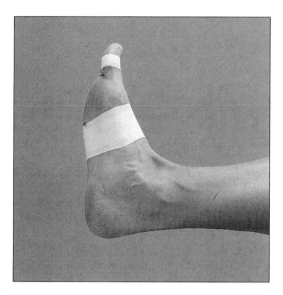

1. *Clean the area and shave dorsum of foot if hairy.*
2. *Spray area with skin toughener or quick-dry adhesive spray to ensure adherence.*

3. *Place an anchor of 2 cm (3/4 in.) white tape around distal toe at base of toenail.*
4. *Place two anchors of 3.8 cm (1.5 in.) white tape around instep and arch of foot.*

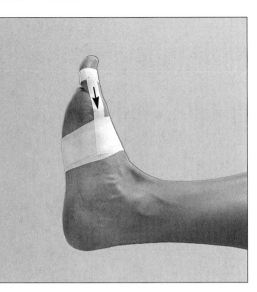

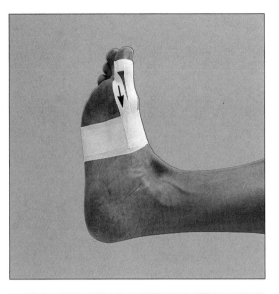

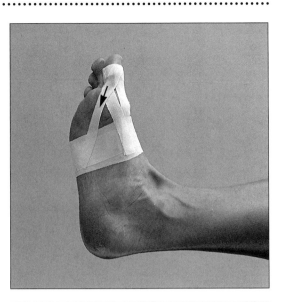

5. *Place a longitudinal supporting strip of 2 cm (3/4 in.) white tape from **distal** to **proximal** anchor on medial aspect of foot.*

NOTE: Abduct the toe slightly and apply 2 strips - with tension - when taping for a medial collateral ligament sprain or for bunions.

6. *Begin a plantar **X** with a longitudinal strip diagonally from **lateral** aspect of distal anchor to medial aspect of **proximal** anchor on plantar aspect of first metatarsophalangeal (MTP) joint.*

7. *Cross this with second strip from the medial aspect of **distal** anchor crossing MTP joint at its midpoint on plantar aspect.*

NOTE: Extension must be adequately limited with this X when taping hyperextension injuries.

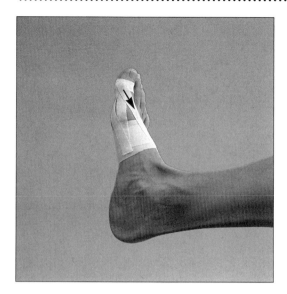

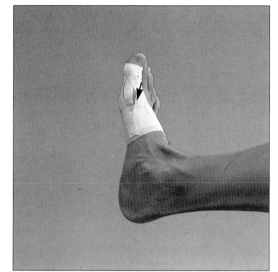

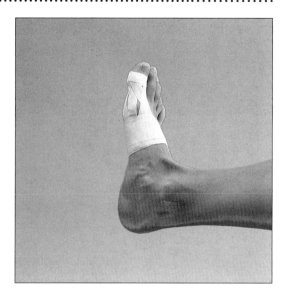

8. *Begin dorsal **X** with a 2 cm (3/4 in.) strip from the medial aspect of the **distal** anchor to dorsal aspect of the proximal anchor.*

9. *Finish the dorsal **X** by crossing this strip from lateral aspect of **distal** anchor to medial aspect of **proximal** anchor, crossing the **X** over dorsal MTP joint.*

NOTE: Flexion must be adequately limited with this X when taping hyperflexion injuries.

10. *Close up taping with light circumferential strips covering sites of original anchors with 2 cm (3/4 in.) and 3.8 cm (1.5 in.) tape, starting proximally and moving distally, overlapping each previous strip by 1/2.*

11. *Test taping for adequate restriction to ensure adequate pain-free functional support.*

NOTE: The colour, temperature and sensation must be checked to verify that circulation has not been compromised.

ANATOMICAL AREA: FOOT AND ANKLE

INJURY: TOE SPRAIN

T ERMINOLOGY:
- sprain of medial or lateral collateral ligament
- hyperflexion with capsular injury
- hyperextension with capsular injury
- sprain of the plantar ligament
- "jammed" toe; "stubbed" toe; "turf" toe.

E TIOLOGY:
- sudden forced flexion, extension or abduction
- sudden longitudinal impact against a hard surface
- repetitive dorsiflexion of great toe (as in kicking a ball or sprinting) can cause a synovitis.
- chronic sprain
- inadequately supportive footwear on artificial turf.

S YMPTOMS:
- tenderness of the first metatarsophalangeal joint
- often swollen
- active movement testing:
  a. pain on end-range flexion with hyperflexion injuries
  b. pain on end-range extension with hyperextension injuries
  c. pain on end-range abduction with medial collateral ligament sprain
- passive movement testing:
  a. pain on end-range flexion with hyperflexion injuries
  b. pain on end-range extension with hyperextension injuries
  c. pain on end-range abduction with medial collateral ligament sprain
- resistance testing (neutral position): no significant pain on moderate resistance
- stress testing:
  a. pain with or without laxity on medial (or lateral) stress with 1st and 2nd degree sprains of the medial (or lateral) collateral ligaments
  b. instability with less pain in 3rd degree sprains

T REATMENT
Early:
- R.I.C.E.S.
- taping for: **Toe Sprain taping,** *see* **page 52**.
- therapeutic modalities

Later:
- continued physiotherapy including:
- therapeutic modalities
- passive mobilizations if painful or stiff
- flexibility
- strengthening exercises
- gradual pain-free reintegration to sports activities with taped support
- a shoe with stiff soles for reinforcement may be necessary.
- dynamic weightbearing activity should start only after 45° of pain-free dorsiflexion is attained.

S EQUELAE:
- pain
- chronic swelling
- diminished mobility
- weakness
- chronic synovitis
- flexor hallucis longus tendinitis
- degenerate changes leading to hallux rigidus (stiff first toe)

R.I.C.E.S. : Rest, Ice, Compress, Elevate, Support

ANATOMICAL AREA: FOOT AND ANKLE

TAPING FOR LONGITUDINAL ARCH SPRAIN / PLANTAR FASCIITIS

Purpose:
- supports plantar aspect of foot (functionally shortens and reinforces the longitudinal arches – medial more than lateral)
- permits plantar flexion mobility
- limits extension (dorsiflexion) of the midtarsal joints

Indications for use:
- plantar fasciitis
- acute or chronic mid foot sprains
- flat feet or fallen arches
- medial knee pain caused by flat feet
- bone spurs
- shin splints

MATERIALS:

razor
skin toughener spray
1.2 cm (1/2 in.) white tape
3.8 cm (1.5 in.) (can be split to make 1 cm (0.4 in.) width)

NOTES:
- Pressure on base of 5th metatarsal bone can cause acute pain.
- Pressure on its neighbouring artery can cause pain and compromise circulation.
- Tape thickness must be kept to a minimum for sports requiring a tight-fitting boot or shoe.
- Excessive medial tension must be avoided, particularly in ankles predisposed to inversion sprains.

For additional details regarding an injury example see TESTS chart page 63

Positioning
Either prone lying with knee slightly bent (as illustrated) or sitting up facing the taper.

Procedure:

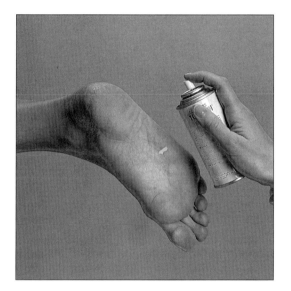

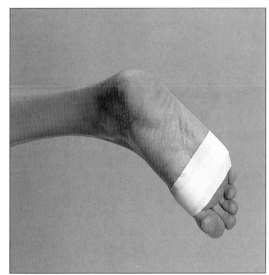

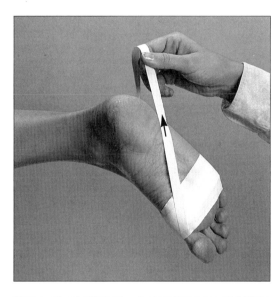

1. *Clean foot and check for skin infections or skin conditions, and signs of chronic inflammatory diseases.*
2. *Shave dorsum of foot if excessively hairy.*
3. *Spray area with skin toughener.*

4. *Place anchor strips of 3.8 cm (1.5 in.) white tape using light tension around the foot at the level of the heads of metatarsals.*

TIP: Allow for some splaying of metatarsals (transverse arch) when applying anchors to avoid discomfort and cramping on subsequent weightbearing.

5a. *Using firm tension, place a strip of 1.2 cm (1/2 in.) white tape from the head of the first metatarsal under the arch around the heel.*

NOTE: 3/4" or 1" tape can be used for larger feet.

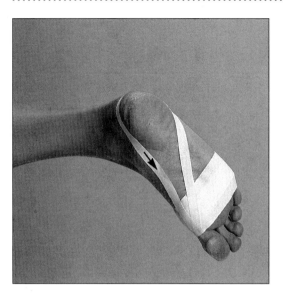

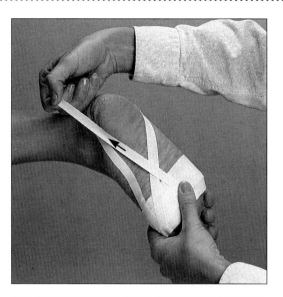

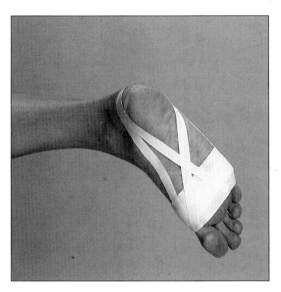

5b. *Finish at the medial aspect of the head of the first metatarsal, shortening the medial arch.*

6a. *Starting from the lateral aspect of the anchor's plantar surface, apply a second strip, with strong tension, crossing the transverse arch diagonally around the heel.*

6b. *Pass behind the heel without tension and finish over the lateral aspect of the head of fifth metatarsal.*

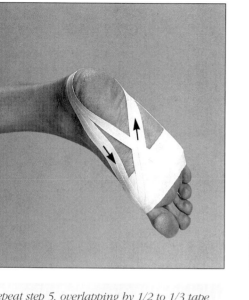

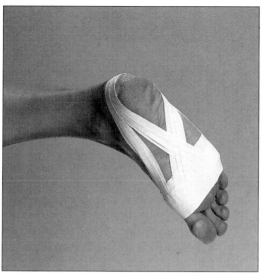

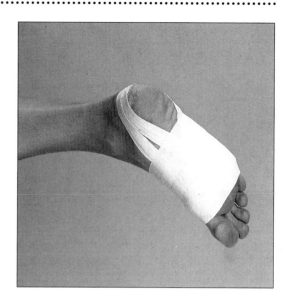

7. Repeat step 5, overlapping by 1/2 to 1/3 tape width moving laterally.

8. Repeat step 6 overlapping by 1/2 to 1/3 tape width, again moving laterally.

9. Repeat steps 5 and 6 overlapping by 1/2 to 1/3 tape width, moving laterally.

10. Close up with circumferential strips of 3.8 cm (1.5 in.) white tape. Apply with firm upwards pressure, following contours of foot with each strip, beginning at the heads of the metatarsals, progressing towards the heel, overlapping strip by 1/3 to 1/2 each progression

11. Test for degree of support. There should be a significant (or complete) reduction of pain on weightbearing.

NOTE: When ankle stability is a concern, a Figure-8 can be added: see steps 12 and 13.

Longitudinal Arch Sprain (plantar fasciitis)

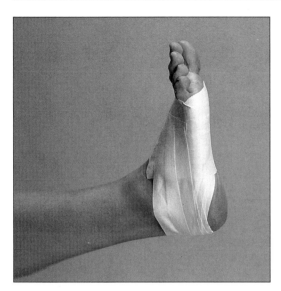

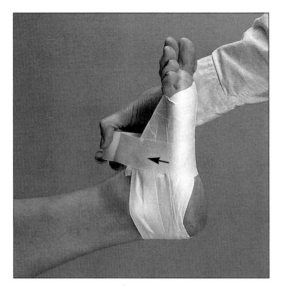

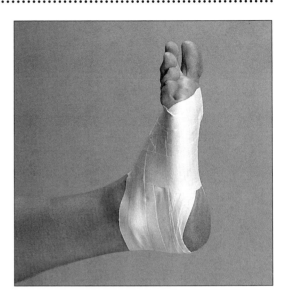

12. *Apply two overlapping horizontal strips of 3.8 cm (1.5 in.) white tape with lubricant.*

NOTE: Apply lubricant and heel and lace pads to the anterior ankle and posterior heel if friction spots are likely to develop.

13a. *Start a figure-8 strip on the dorsum (top) of the foot from lateral to medial. Pass under the arch and pull up strongly on the lateral side of the foot.*

13b. *Continue around behind the heel and complete the figure-8 anteriorly.*

NOTE: This strip can be repeated with a slight overlap to reinforce lateral stability.

ANATOMICAL AREA: FOOT AND ANKLE

CONDITION: PLANTAR FASCIITIS

T ERMINOLOGY:
- chronic or acute inflammation of plantar fascia
- heel spurs

E TIOLOGY
- intrinsically tight plantar fascia
- poor foot biomechanics
- sudden change in training routine: i.e. distance, frequency, speed, change of terrain
- poorly supportive or new footwear
- secondary to mid-foot sprain or tarsal hypomobility

S YMPTOMS:
- pain and tenderness on plantar aspect of foot: more concentrated on the medial aspect of calcaneal attachment
- active movement testing: no significant pain non weightbearing
- passive movement testing: pain on full stretch of fascia
- resistance testing (neutral position): no significant pain
- pain on first steps after resting
- pain on weightbearing: particularly on push-off

T REATMENT:
- physiotherapy including:
- R.I.C.E.S.
- therapeutic modalities (use of laser or ultrasound can be particularly helpful)
- Support: taping: **Longitudinal Arch Taping:** *see* **page 58**.
- Rest: reduction of weightbearing activities
- selective stretching to tendo-Achilles and of plantar fascia
- strengthening of plantar muscles
- heel lifts can be helpful in acute phase
  (a bevelled donut depression will reduce pressure pain)

S EQUELAE:
- injury often becomes chronic without correct treatment
- development of heel spurs
- tight tendo-Achilles complex
- may predispose to shin splints
- orthotics may be indicated

R.I.C.E.S. : Rest, Ice, Compress, Elevate, Support

Longitudinal Arch Sprain (plantar fasciitis)

ANATOMICAL AREA: FOOT AND ANKLE

TAPING FOR: PREVENTATIVE PROPHYLACTIC ANKLE SPRAINS

MATERIALS:

razor
skin toughener spray
lubricant
heel and lace pads
prowrap
3.8 cm (1.5 in.) white tape

Purpose:
- offers bilateral ankle stability with specific reinforcement of the lateral ligaments.
- restricts inversion and some eversion.
- allows almost full range of dorsiflexion and plantar flexion.

Indications for use:
- preventative taping to protect: 1) lax ligaments and 2) "weak" ankles
- final stages of ankle sprain rehabilitation, when less specific ligamentous reinforcement is sufficient.
- chronic inversion sprains
- for chronic medial sprains (deltoid ligament): reverse strips (steps 6–8 and 10–12, 14 and 16) to reinforce medial rather than lateral support.

NOTES:
- It is essential to confirm the site of the original injury prior to taping, so that specific reinforcement can be made either medially or laterally.
- The athlete should be queried as to whether a very restrictive or light taping is preferable. Tension can be adjusted to suit individual preference during the procedure.
- Pressure over the base of the fifth metatarsal bone can cause acute pain; pressure on its neighbouring artery can cause pain and compromise circulation.
- Ankles are prone to re-spraining for as long as one year after the original injury. (It takes at least 12 months for a severely sprained ligament to regain its tensile strength.)
- Proprioception retraining is extremely important to ensure a total recovery program.

For additional details regarding an injury example see TESTS chart page 88.

Positioning:

Lying supine (face up) or long-sitting (knees extended) with the ankle held at a 90° angle over the end of the table and supported at the mid-calf.

TIP: The taping surface should be high enough that the taper can work comfortably without risking back strain.

Procedure:

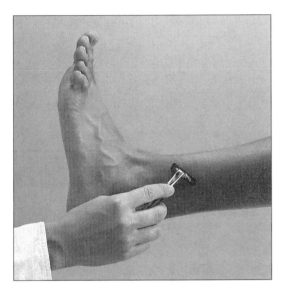

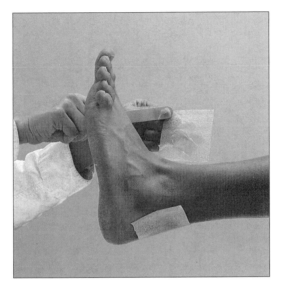

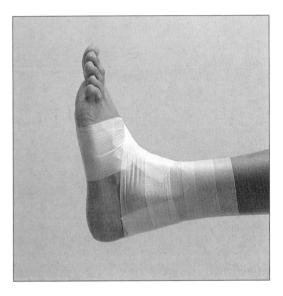

1. *Ensure that the area to be taped is clean, shaved and dry.*
2. *Check skin for cuts, blisters or irritated areas before spraying with skin toughener.*

3. *Apply lubricated heel and lace pads to the two "danger" areas where blisters or tape cuts frequently occur.*

4. *Apply prowrap to area to be taped.*

TIP: Cover the Achilles tendon including its attachment to the heel and the superficial extensor tendons at the front of the ankle.

Ankle Sprain (preventative)

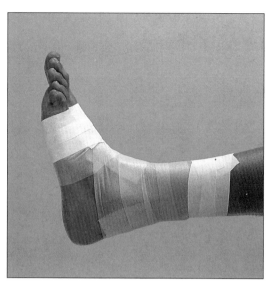

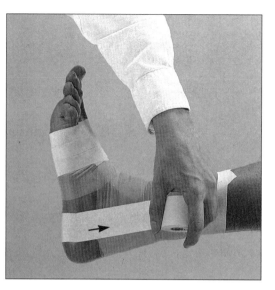

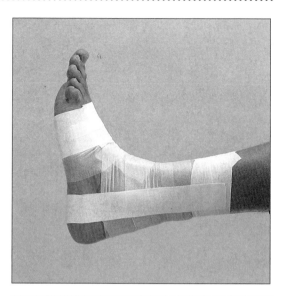

5. *Using light tension, apply two overlapping, circumferential anchor strips of 3.8 cm (1.5 in.) white tape at the forefoot and two below the calf bulk (at the musculotendinous junction).*

TIP: When applying the anchor strips mid-calf, be sure that the strip is held horizontally at the back and wraps around the natural contours rising up to cross more superiorly on the anterior surface.

NOTE: These anchors must be in direct contact with the skin to ensure support.

6. *Apply a stirrup of 3.8 cm (1.5 in.) white tape . Starting from the upper anchor medially, pass under the heel and pull up with tension ending on the upper anchor laterally .*

TIP: Be sure the ankle is kept at a 90° angle throughout this procedure.

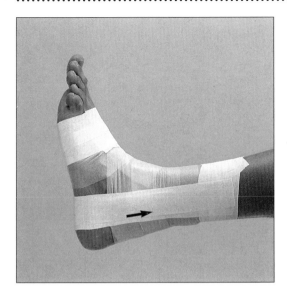

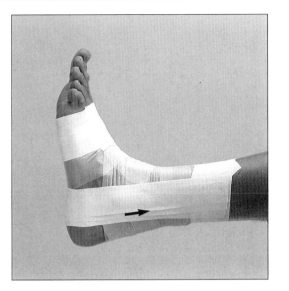

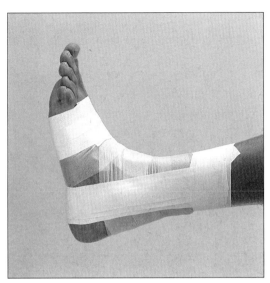

7. *Apply a second stirrup, beginning and ending more anteriorly.*

8. *Apply a third stirrup beginning and ending more anteriorly.*

9. *Repeat the proximal anchor (5).*

TIP: Always pull up strongly on the lateral side.

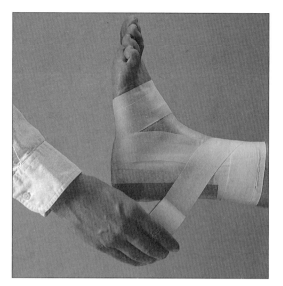

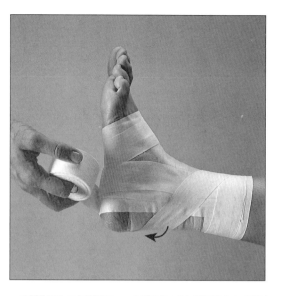

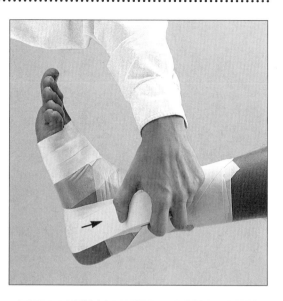

10. Apply the first ankle-lock:
a. Beginning on the anterior shin, pass towards the lateral aspect of the ankle,

10b. Continue cautiously behind the Achilles tendon, around and under the heel.

10c. Pull up over the lateral side applying strong tension and fix securely to the lateral upper anchor.

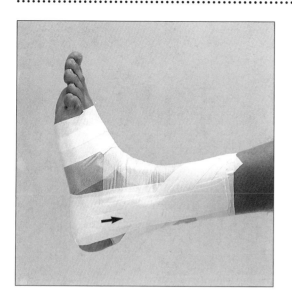

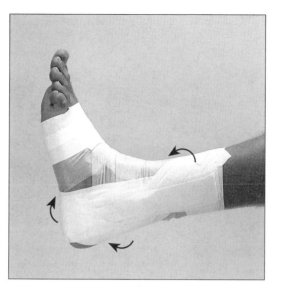

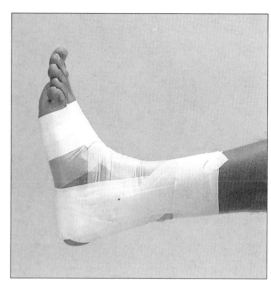

11. *Repeat this lateral ankle lock (step 10) once more .*

12. *Apply a medial ankle lock by reversing this strip starting and finishing on the medial side for added stability.*

TIP: Apply medium tension only when pulling up on the medial side.

13. *Begin closing up the tape job from the top ensuring all gaps ('windows') are covered in order to avoid blisters.*

NOTE: By overlapping the tape strips from top to bottom, the tape will not catch and tend to roll back as the athlete pulls on his socks.

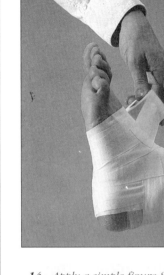 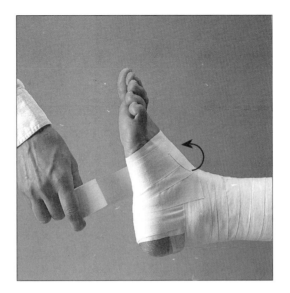 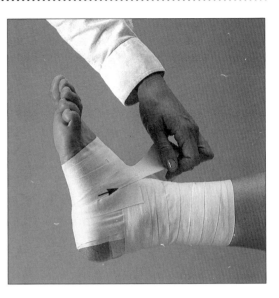

14. *Apply a simple figure-8 to close and to reinforce the ankle:*

   a. *Start anteriorly crossing medially without tension.*

14b. *Pull the tape down towards the medial aspect of the arch,*

14c. *Pass under the foot and pull up with firm tension over the lateral side before crossing the ankle anteriorly with less tension.*

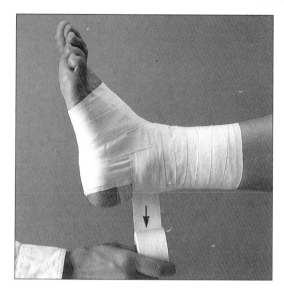

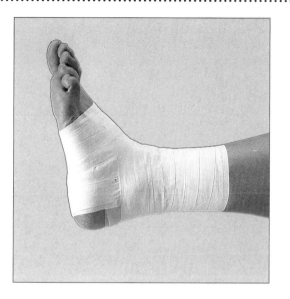

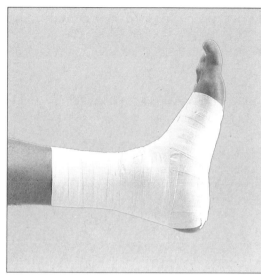

14d. *Bring the tape horizontally behind the Achilles tendon and finish anteriorly, crossing the starting point of this strip.*

> **NOTE:** a second figure-8 can be applied to offer greater support or to cover any remaining open areas.

15. *Complete the closing up strips covering the forefoot if not already completely closed in.*

16. *Test the degree of restriction.*
a. *Inversion should be significantly restricted*
b. *Plantar flexion should be limited by 30° or more.*

> **NOTE:** Medial view of finished tape job is shown in this photo.

ANATOMICAL AREA: FOOT AND ANKLE

TAPING FOR: ANKLE SPRAIN/CONTUSION: ACUTE STAGE

Purpose:
- gives lateral stability through splinting and compression
- permits some plantar flexion and dorsiflexion
- controls swelling without compromising arterial and nerve supply (removal of the safety strip permits easy release of tension in case of progressive swelling)

Indications for use:
- acute (inversion) lateral ankle sprain
- acute (eversion) medial ankle sprains: reverse strips 5, 9, 12, 19, and 20 to support medially damaged structures
- acute post-cast removal
- splinting for suspected ankle fracture: use less tension and apply equally to both sides
- acute ankle contusion: apply tension to injured side

MATERIALS:

razor
skin toughener spray
3.8 cm (1.5 in.) white tape
felt or foam cut into a
horseshoe or "J" shape
7.5 cm (3 in.) elastic wrap

NOTES:
- Ensure that a correct diagnosis is made:
  a. a fracture may be suspected particularly if the athlete is unable to bear weight.
  b. X-rays should be obtained even in less painful cases in order to rule out an avulsion fracture.
  c. stress testing of the ligaments will indicate localization and severity of sprain.
- Care must be taken to apply adequate, localized compression over the basic taping without compromising the circulation. Too much circumferential tension will cause a tourniquet effect.
- Ensure that the athlete has been thoroughly instructed in the care of the injured ankle: first 48 hours post-injury: R.I.C.E.S. (Rest, Ice, Compress, Elevate, Support)
- Watch for numbness, swelling or cyanosis (blueish colouring) of the toes.
- Should the taping become too tight due to uncontrollable swelling (even when ice has been used and the ankle elevated), the anterior safety strip must be removed or loosened and the compression re-applied.

For additional details regarding an injury example see TESTS chart page 88.

Positioning:

Lying supine (face up) with a cushioned support under the mid-calf and with the injured ankle held at 90°.

Procedure:

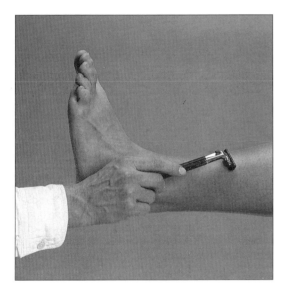

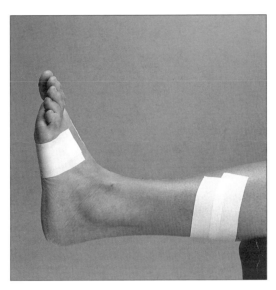

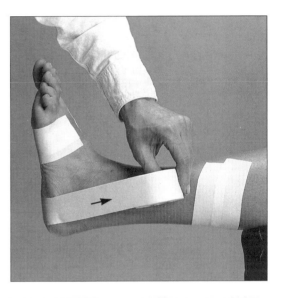

1. *Clean, shave and dry the area to be taped, checking for cuts, abrasions or sensitive skin.*

2. *Spray the area with skin toughener or quick dry adhesive to protect the skin from irritation and to ensure good adhesion.*

3. *Apply two open anchors of 3.8 cm (1.5 in.) white tape around lower third of calf. Be sure to leave an open space in front.*

> TIP: Ensure that these anchors are horizontal in the back of the calf, and lie evenly across the front of the shin.

4. *Apply two anchors around the midfoot, leaving an open space on the dorsum (top).*

5. *Apply a stirrup of 3.8 cm (1.5 in.) from the medial upper anchor down the medial side, passing beneath the heel, and slightly behind the lateral malleolus. Pull up strongly to apply specific tension over the lateral side.*

> NOTE: When taping MEDIALLY injured structures, this strip is started on the LATERAL side and pulled up strongly on the MEDIAL side for reinforcement. Also in steps 9 and 12.

Ankle Sprain (acute)

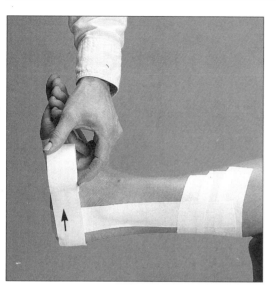

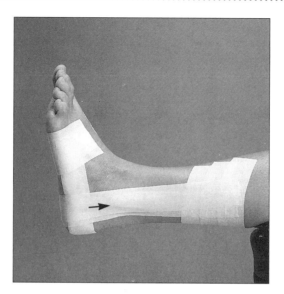

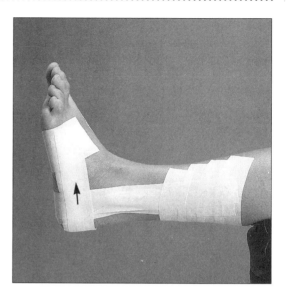

6. Apply an open anchor around the upper end of this stirrup overlapping the original anchor by 1/3 inferiorly.

7. Apply a horizontal strip at the level of the tip of the lateral malleolus putting extra tension on the lateral side.

8. Stabilize this horizontal strip with a vertical forefoot anchor overlapping the previous anchor by 1/2.

9. Apply a second stirrup as in step 5 overlapping the previous stirrup by 2/3 anteriorly.

10. Anchor the stirrup as in Step 6 moving lower on the calf covering the previous anchor by 1/3.

11. Apply a horizontal strip overlapping the previous strip by 1/2, pulling strongly on the lateral side.

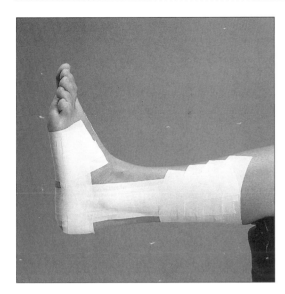

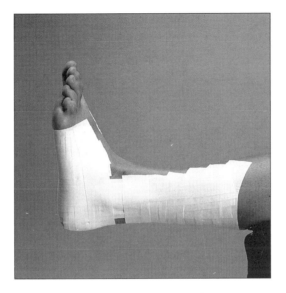

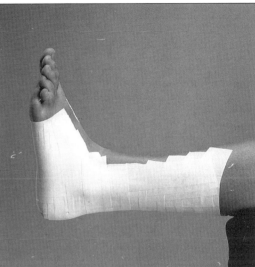

12. *Repeat steps 8 & 9 overlapping the previous strips always pulling strongly on the lateral side.*

13. *Repeat steps 10 & 11 overlapping again in the same manner.*

14. *Repeat steps 8–11 until all gaps in the taping have been covered.*

TIP: Be sure the ankle is kept at a 90° angle throughout this procedure.

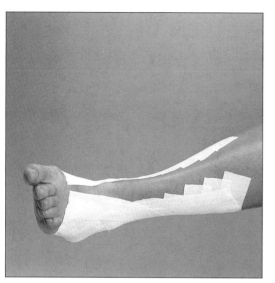

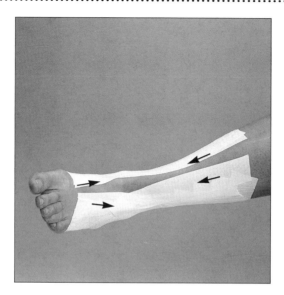

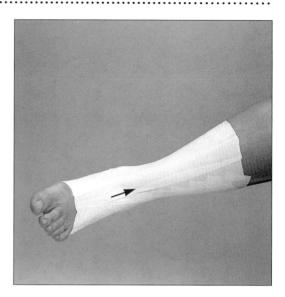

15. *Apply a pair of vertical strips lightly covering the tape ends on either side of the gap anteriorly from the shin to the ankle.*
16. *Apply a second pair of parallel strips from the forefoot, pulling up slightly and covering the previous strip at the ankle.*
17. *Gently test the degree of restriction:*
  a. *there must be no laxity on lateral stress testing*
  b. *there should be significantly reduced pain if any on passive inversion and eversion. Add reinforcements if necessary.*

18. *Apply a final single safety strip to close off the remaining open area.*

TIP: Allow slight plantar flexion while applying this strip to ensure continuous adhesion of the tape at the front of the ankle.

NOTE: This safety strip is easily loosened in case of progressive swelling.

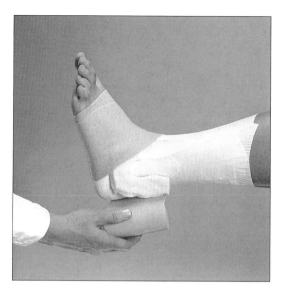

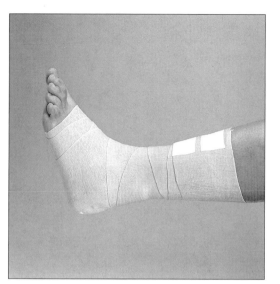

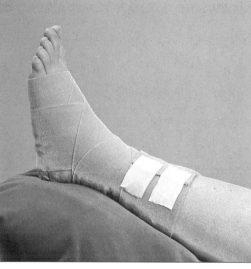

19. *For added control of swelling, cut a felt or dense foam pad in the shape of a "J" or a horseshoe to fill the hollows around the lateral malleolus (ankle bone). (Bevel the edges.)*

20a. *Apply an elastic bandage to hold it in place using a figure-8 pattern.*

20b. *Stretch the elastic wrap each time as it crosses the lateral side and relax the tension while covering the medial side. Continue, with gradually diminishing tension, until the bandage covers the entire tape job.*

21. *Elevate the injury for the first 48 hours.*

TIP: Luggage can be placed underneath the mattress to elevate the foot of the bed if an appropriate bolster is not available

NOTE: THIS IS NOT A WEIGHTBEARING TAPE JOB.

ANATOMICAL AREA: FOOT AND ANKLE

TAPING FOR LATERAL ANKLE SPRAIN: REHABILITATION STAGE

Purpose:
- offers lateral stability with specific reinforcement
- prevents inversion
- restricts end-range plantar flexion and some eversion
- allows almost full dorsiflexion and functional plantar flexion

Indications for use:
- lateral ankle sprains (INVERSION sprain)
- injuries of the calcaneo-fibular and the anterior talo-fibular ligaments: in combination, the most common ankle sprain.
- for medial ankle sprains (deltoid ligament): use a horseshoe instead of a "J" shape on the medial side in step 6 and reverse steps 9–11 and 15–16 for medial instead of lateral reinforcement.

MATERIALS

razor
skin toughener spray
prowrap
3.8 cm (1.5 in.) white tape
2 cm (3/4 in.) felt or foam cut into a horseshoe or "J" shape
2 cm (3/4 in.) felt heel lift
7.5 cm (3 in.) elastic wrap for small ankles
10 cm (4 in.) for large ankles

NOTES:
- Ensure that the injury has been properly evaluated by a competent sports medicine specialist, and that X-rays have been taken particularly if an avulsion fracture is suspected.
- DO NOT USE THIS TECHNIQUE IF THIS IS AN ACUTE ANKLE INJURY. It should only be applied when acute swelling has subsided. (For Acute Ankle Injury taping see page 72)
- Placement of a felt horseshoe controls residual peri-malleolar swelling - particularly useful in the sub-acute phase when localized swelling can become chronic.
- PWB (partial weightbearing) with crutches is recommended when starting to weightbear.
- Progression to FWB (full weightbearing) is permitted only if pain-free.
- Use of a heel lift assists "push-off" and reduces the need for dorsiflexion range, allowing weightbearing with less effort and stress.
- Weightbearing activities may be continued and progressed only if there is no pain **during** or **after** activity.

Taping is adapted throughout the progressive rehabilitation healing stages:

1. **sub-acute stage:** (after 48 hours post-injury): support with felt J and heel lift while beginning to weightbear.
2. **functional stage:** specific ligamentous support with reinforcement of stability for moderate to dynamic activity.
3. **return to sport stage:** reintegration with support adapted to specific sports requirements ranging from training to competition.

For additional details regarding an injury example see TESTS chart page 88.

Positioning:

Lying supine (face up) or long-sitting (sitting with knees extended) support at mid calf with the foot off the end of the table. The ankle must be held at a 90° angle throughout the taping.

Procedure:

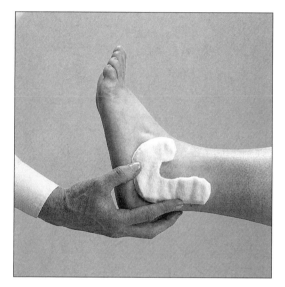

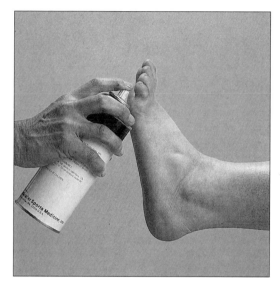

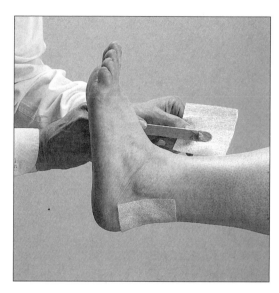

1. *Ensure that the area to be taped is clean, shaved and dry.*
2. *To control swelling, cut a felt or dense foam pad in the shape of a "J" or a horseshoe to fill the hollows around the malleolus (ankle bone). Bevel the edges of the pad to form fit all the contours.*

TIP: Keep this felt shape within handy reach, ready to apply.

3. *Check skin for cuts, blisters or irritated areas before spraying with skin toughener.*

4. *If repetitive activity is to be undertaken, apply lubricated heel and lace pads to the two "danger" areas where blisters or tape cuts frequently occur.*

Ankle Sprain Rehabilitation (basic)

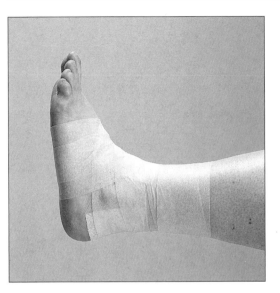

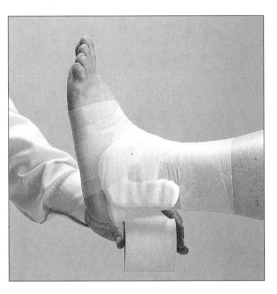

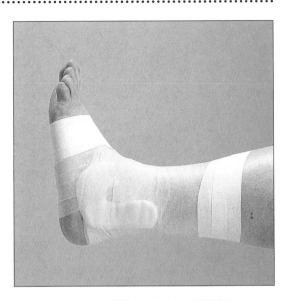

5. *Apply prowrap to area to be taped.*

6. *Attach the felt piece with a figure-8 of prowrap.*

TIP: By placing the felt horseshoe between two layers of prowrap, it can be retrieved easily when the tape is removed. (This adapted "horseshoe" can then be reused when the tape job is renewed, saving time, energy and expense.)

7. *Using light tension, apply two overlapping, circumferential anchor strips of 3.8 cm (1.5 in.) white tape below the calf bulk at the musculotendinous junction.*

TIP: Start each strip horizontally at the back and follow the natural contour of the leg, rising up to overlap higher on the anterior surface.

8. *Apply two overlapping anchor strips around the forefoot.*

TIP: Allow for some splaying of the metatarsals to avoid discomfort when subjected to weightbearing.

NOTE: These anchors must be in direct contact with the skin to ensure support.

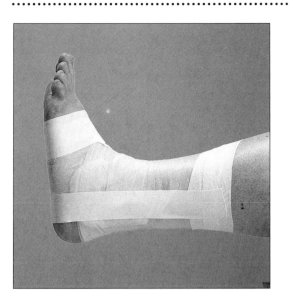

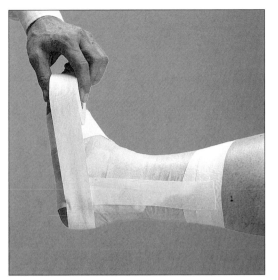

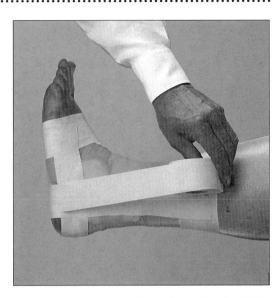

9. *Apply a stirrup of 3.8 cm (1.5 in.) white tape starting from the upper anchor medially. Cover the posterior edge of the medial malleolus, pass beneath the heel, and up, covering the posterior edge of the malleolus. Pull up strongly to apply specific tension over the lateral side and affix the tape to the upper anchor laterally.*

10. *Starting on the medial side of the distal anchor, apply a horizontal strip passing behind the heel and covering the tip of the lateral malleolus. Put extra tension on the lateral side before reattaching the tape to the distal anchor on its lateral side.*

11. *Apply a second stirrup as in step 9, overlapping the previous stirrup by 2/3, anteriorly.*

TIP:
- Ensure that the ankle is kept at a 90° angle throughout this procedure.
- Apply strong tension up the lateral side.

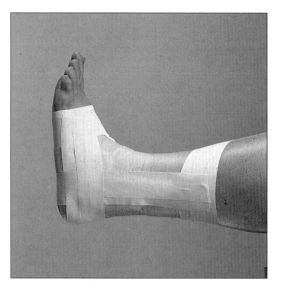

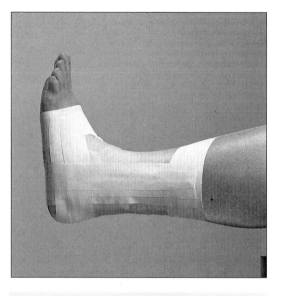

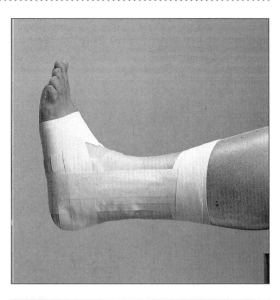

12. *Apply a second horizontal strip as in strip 10, overlapping the previous strip by 1/2 superiorly, covering the malleoli.*

TIP: Always apply specific tension on the lateral side.

13. *Apply a third stirrup as in step 9, overlapping the previous stirrup by 2/3 anteriorly.*

NOTE:
- A third horizontal strip may be necessary when taping large feet and when additional horizontal stability is required.
- These stirrups may be "fanned" when the athlete is at the returning to sport stage of rehabilitation. (See Fanned Stirrups, page 90).

14. *Repeat the proximal and distal anchors.*

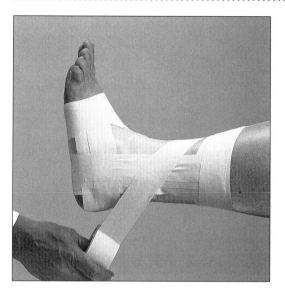

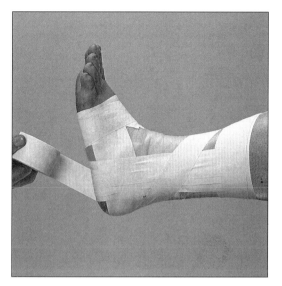

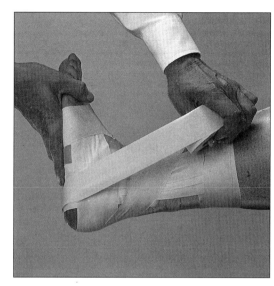

15. *Apply the first lateral ankle lock:*
a. *begin on the anterior shin passing towards the lateral aspect of the ankle,*

15b. *continue behind the Achilles tendon, around and under the heel,*

15c. *then apply strong tension up over the lateral side to the lateral upper anchor.*

NOTE: Be careful to start with the appropriate angle so that the tape will follow the contours and end up in the appropriate place.

TIP: Support and hold the foot in eversion (turned outward) to ensure a shortened position for the ligaments while applying this important supporting strip.

Ankle Sprain Rehabilitation (basic)

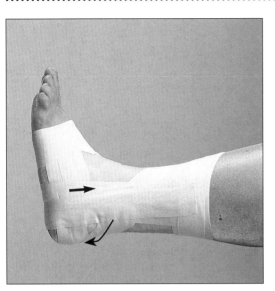

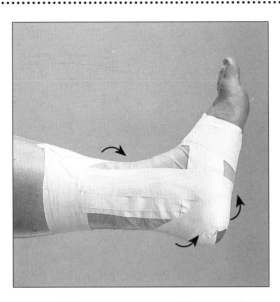

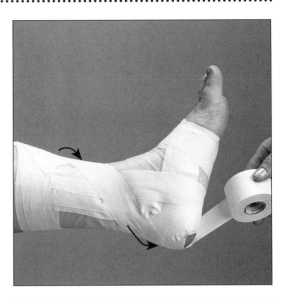

16. *Repeat step 15 again on the lateral side overlapping the previous strip by 3/4.*

View from the medial side.

17a. *To balance stability, apply the ankle lock once on the medial side.*

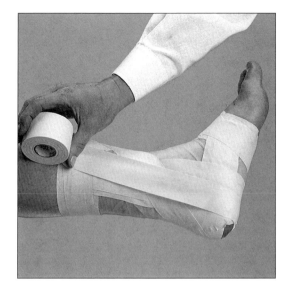

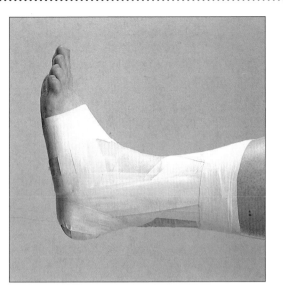

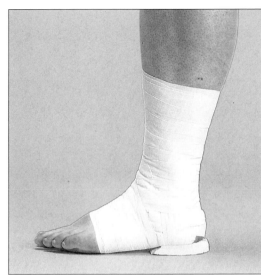

17b. *Less tension when pulling up on the medial side.*

18. *Reanchor proximally.*

19. *Close up the tape job by starting proximally (at the top and progressing distally (downwards) overlapping each previous strip by 1/3 to 1/2 its width, ensuring all gaps ("windows") are covered in order to avoid blisters.*

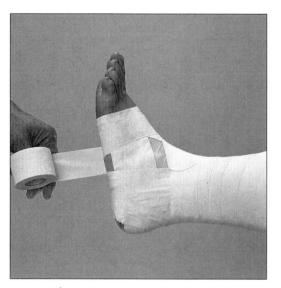

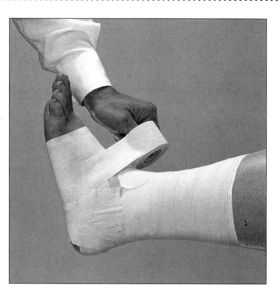

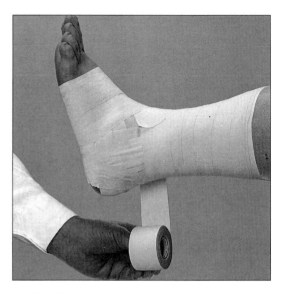

20. *Apply a simple figure-8 to close and to reinforce the ankle:*

a. *Start anteriorly crossing the ankle towards the medial aspect of the midfoot and pass under the foot,*

20b. *pulling up with firm tension over the lateral side before crossing the ankle anteriorly with less tension.*

20c. *Bring the tape horizontally behind the Achilles tendon.*

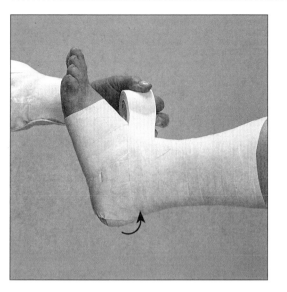

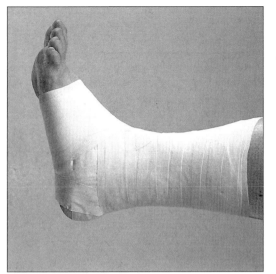

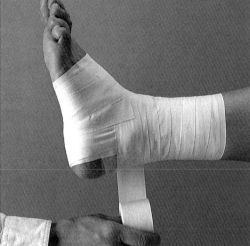

20d. *Finish anteriorly, crossing the starting point of the strip.*

TIP: Apply a second figure-8 if necessary to cover any open areas (overlap the first figure-8 by 1/2).

NOTE: For return to dynamic activity, a heel-locking figure-8 (see page 94) or a reverse figure-8 (see page 96) can be applied in place of the regular figure-8.

21. *Complete the closing-up strips covering the forefoot and distal anchors.*
22. *Gently at first, test the degree of inversion and plantar flexion restricted by the tape. Add reinforcements if these movements are not adequately limited or if they cause pain.*

TIP: A 1/2 in. heel lift (bevelled at the front edge) will raise the heel and reduce stress on the injured ligaments. Particularly useful during the subacute stage when weightbearing commences.

NOTE: Weightbearing and gradually increasing activity must only be permitted if pain-free, both during and after activity.

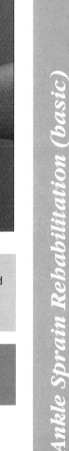

Ankle Sprain Rehabilitation (basic)

ANATOMICAL AREA: FOOT AND ANKLE

INJURY: LATERAL ANKLE SPRAIN
(typically a combination of two ligaments: calcaneo-fibular and anterior talo-fibular)

T ERMINOLOGY:
- **see sprains chart page 36 degree of severity.**
- inversion sprain
- "turned" ankle

E TIOLOGY:
- forced inversion with plantar flexion;
- "rolling-over" on ankle
- often secondary to inadequate rehabilitation of a previous ankle sprain (reduced proprioception)
- the **MOST** commonly injured combination of ankle ligaments.

S YMPTOMS:
- local pain, swelling, discolouration and tenderness anteriorly and inferior to the lateral malleolus.
- active movement testing: pain on plantar flexion with inversion
- passive movement testing: pain on plantar flexion with inversion
- resistance testing (neutral position): no significant pattern of pain with moderate resistance
- stress testing:
  a. pain, with or without laxity, on anterior "drawer" test (forward gliding of the talus under the tibio-fibular mortice) indicates a 1st or 2nd degree sprain of the anterior talo-fibular ligament.
  b. instability on forward displacement of the talus away from the lateral malleolus indicates a 3rd degree sprain of the same ligament.
  c. pain with or without some laxity on talar tilt test indicates a 1st or 2nd degree sprain of the fibulo-calcaneal.
  d. instability or "opening up" on the talar tilt test (often with little or no pain) is indicative of a 3rd degree sprain of this ligament.

T REATMENT:
Early:
- R.I.C.E.S.
- taping: first 48 hours: **Acute Ankle Injury (open basketweave) see page 72.**
- therapeutic modalities

Later:
- continued physiotherapy including:
  - therapeutic modalities
  - transverse friction massage
  - modified fitness activities
  - progressive pain-free rehabilitation including:
  a. range of motion
  b. flexibility
  c. strength: non-weightbearing to weightbearing (endurance, then power)
  d. proprioception
- gradual painfree reintegration to sports activity with specific taping. **(For Ankle Rehabilitation Taping see page 78.)**
- prevention of recurrent sprains

S EQUELAE:
- anterior talo-crural and sub-talar instability if ligaments are not supported in a shortened position during healing phase
- weakness and/or tendinitis of peroneal muscles
- extensor digitorum longus is often injured simultaneously predisposing to chronic residual weakness
- reduced proprioception
- repeated injury caused by poor proprioception and joint instability
- chronic swelling in the sinus tarsi and around the tip of the lateral malleolus.

R.I.C.E.S. : Rest, Ice, Compress, Elevate, Support

ANKLE SPRAIN REHABILITATION – ADVANCED

SPECIAL ADAPTATIONS: Sport-specific ankle taping variations

During the sub-acute and rehabilitation stage of ankle sprains, the tape job is adapted to the varying needs of the injury. Each tape job must be adjusted for the anatomy of the specific ligament, the degree of injury and the current stage of healing. As the athlete gradually returns to sports activity, his sport-specific requirements must also be accommodated.

NOTE: Prior to initial applications of ankle rehabilitation taping strategies, the ankle must be fully evaluated by a competent sports medicine specialist in order to identify the injured structures and to ensure that no other complications exist.

THE FOLLOWING SPECIALIZED STRIP ADAPTATIONS MAY BE USED IN COMBINATION WITH THE PREVIOUSLY DESCRIBED STRIPS TO ADAPT TO A WIDE RANGE OF SITUATIONS BY THE EXPERIENCED TAPER.

Specialized strips for sports-specific techniques include:

- **fanned stirrups:** allows freer plantar flexion (useful when tight boots are required for a specific sports activity).
- **V-lock:** for extra heel stability (useful when the number of tape strips must be kept to a minimum: i.e., when the athlete must wear tight boots).
- **heel-locking figure 8:** reinforces stability when the level of recovery permits a return to activity.
- **reverse figure-8:** reinforces stability without restricting plantar flexion (useful when plantar flexion is needed for sports participation).

SPECIALIZED STRIP: Fanned Stirrups

Purpose:
- offers lateral support over three angles
- useful when tight-fitting footwear is required as in figure-skating, ice hockey, speed-skating and downhill skiing where tape thickness over the malleoli (ankle bones) must be kept to a minimum.

Advantages:
- allows more plantar flexion than straight basketweave stirrups
- mimics multi-angled ligamentous support
- allows minimal tape thickness over bony prominences

Disadvantages:
- reduced limitation of plantar flexion
- thickness is localized under heel

Procedure:

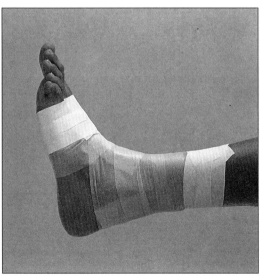

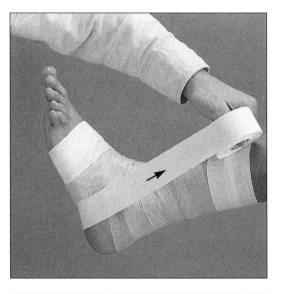

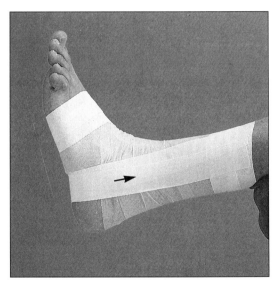

1. *Begin taping by applying steps 1-8 (step 6 is optional) of* **Ankle Rehabilitation taping: page 78.**

2. *Apply the first stirrup starting from the upper anchor posteriorly on the medial side, passing under the heel, and pulling up with a strong tension on the finish more anteriorly on the lateral side of the anchor.*

3. *Attach the second stirrup passing directly over the medial malleolus, passing under the heel and pulling up again with strong tension over the lateral malleolus to the anchor ending slightly posterior than the first stirrup.*

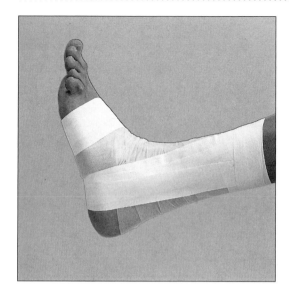

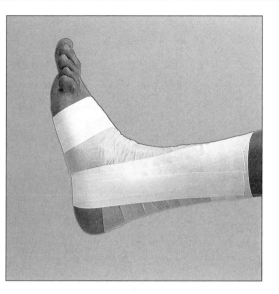

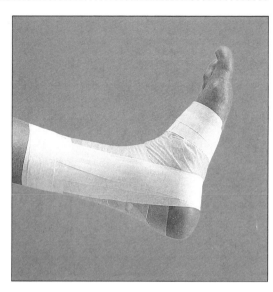

4. *Apply the third stirrup starting more anteriorly on the medial side and finishing posterior to the lateral malleolus on the lateral side.*

TIP: Ensure that strong tension is used when pulling up on the lateral side for all three strips.

5. *Re-anchor these stirrups proximally (at the top) and* **proceed to the complete tape job as in steps 15–22 of Ankle Rehabilitation taping; page 78.**

View from the side

NOTE: These stirrups can be applied in combination with the horizontal strips to form a modified basketweave offering more stable support – particularly for anterior and posterior (talo-fibular or deltoid) ligament sprains.

SPECIALIZED STRIP: V-Lock

Purpose:
- reinforces lateral stability
- locks the heel
- useful when tight-fitting footwear is required, as in figure-skating, ice hockey, speed-skating and downhill skiing where tape thickness over the malleoli (ankle bones) must be kept to a minimum.

Advantages:
- offers a combination of lateral stability and and heel-locking with one single strip.

Disadvantages:
- does not restrict talar tilt as effectively as the single ankle lock.

Procedure:

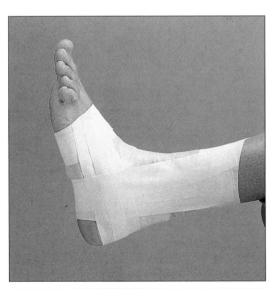

1. *Begin taping by applying steps 1–8 (step 6 is optional) of* **Ankle Rehabilitation taping: page 78.**
   (Fanned stirrups may also be used)

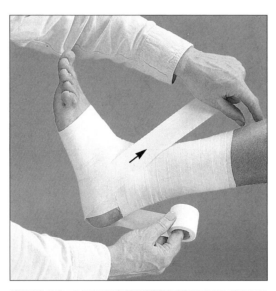

2. *Place the tape under the heel before pulling up on the anterior end and affixing it to the upper anchor, anteriorly.*

TIP: Ensure that the foot is everted (pulled outward) by the pull of this step.

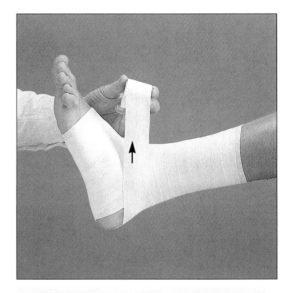

3. *Gently wrap the roll of tape behind the heel, crossing low enough on the lateral side to cover the lateral malleolus.*

4. *Pull the tape snugly across the lateral malleolus to the dorsum of the foot.*

TIP: Lateral shearing of the tape and careful attention to the "take-off" direction will help in achieving the best taping "line" without wrinkling the tape.

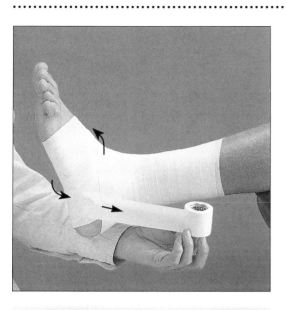

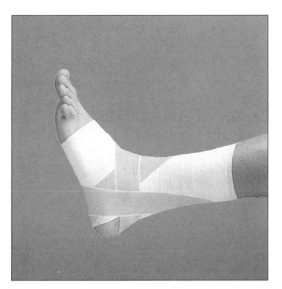

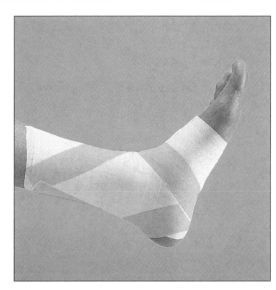

5. *Wrap the tape – without tension – across the front of the ankle*
6. *pass medially to the plantar (inferior) surface under the arch going in a posterior direction.*
7. *Now pull up strongly, posterior to the lateral malleolus, and adhere the strip to the anchor.*

8. *View from the lateral side.*

TIP: Repeated applications using a practice tape strip will improve technique. (See page 40 for preparation of practice strips.)

9. *View from the medial side.*

NOTE: This strip can also be applied to the medial side for added stability and heel-locking effect. Care must be taken not to allow inversion of the ankle when taping for lateral sprains.

Ankle Sprain Rehabilitation (advanced)

SPECIALIZED STRIP: Heel-Locking Figure-8

Procedure:

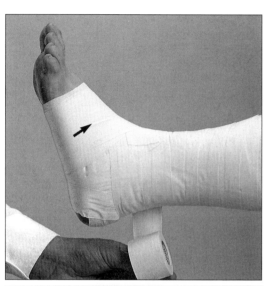

1. *Begin taping by applying steps 1–5, 7–14 of **Ankle Rehabilitation taping, page 78.** (Fanned stirrups may also be used if desired.)*
2. *Start strip on the dorsum of the foot, from lateral to medial, pass under the instep, and pull up strongly on the lateral side.*
3. *Carefully cross the tape over the extensor tendons (without wrinkling) and pass horizontally behind the medial side to wrap around the Achilles tendon.*

TIP: Ensure that the tape is high enough at the back so that the tape is at the same level when it crosses itself again anteriorly.

Purpose:
- offers added reinforcement with specific heel stabilization
- restricts full plantar flexion
- limits lateral mobility
- allows almost full dorsiflexion

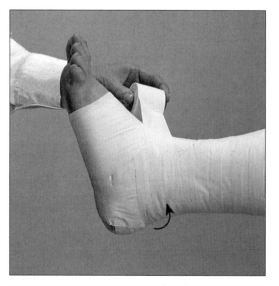

4. *Cross the ankle anteriorly, moving down the medial side and under the instep, slightly posterior to the starting point. Angle the tape in a posterior direction under the plantar surface.*

TIP: The ankle must be adequately dorsiflexed in order to have the tape pass posteriorly without bending, wrinkling, or causing a pressure ridge.

Advantages
- useful in sports requiring more dorsiflexion and where there is less demand for extreme plantar flexion.

Disadvantages:
- restricts plantar flexion

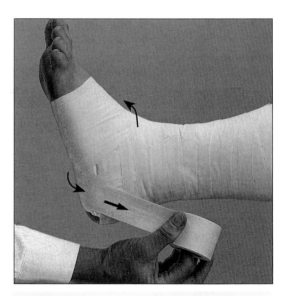

5. *Pull the tape up and back with strong tension posterior to the lateral malleolus and pass behind the Achilles tendon.*

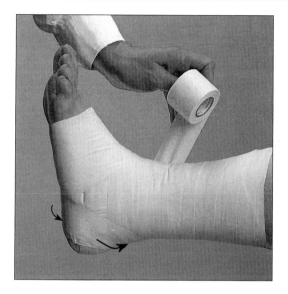

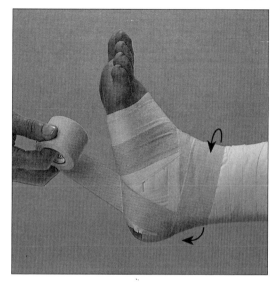

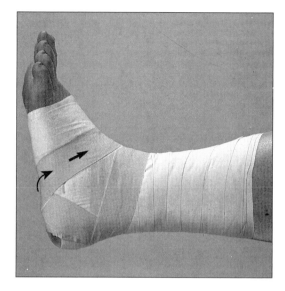

6. *Continue carefully around the front of the ankle.*

TIP: Repeated application using a practice strip will aid in judging taping angles and will improve proficiency significantly. (See page 40 for preparation of practice strips.)

7. *Return posteriorly behind the Achilles tendon again, this time crossing the heel from the medial side and with less tension under the instep.*

8. *Pull up strongly on the lateral side to end by crossing the previous strips anteriorly.*

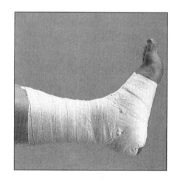

View from the medial side.

SPECIALIZED STRIP: Reverse Figure-8

Purpose:
- offers added reinforcement with specific heel stabilization to a taped ankle.
- restricts dorsiflexion
- limits lateral mobility of ankle and controls heel
- allows almost full plantar flexion

Advantages:
- as this strip allows plantar flexion, it is particularly useful in sports that require a greater functional range of plantar flexion (basketball, volleyball, gymnastics, various track and field sports)
- controls heel from both sides

Disadvantages:
- less stable in plantar flexion than offered by the other figure-8 strips.

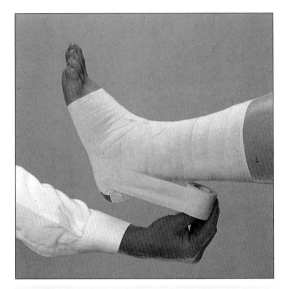

Procedure:

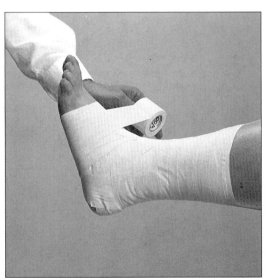

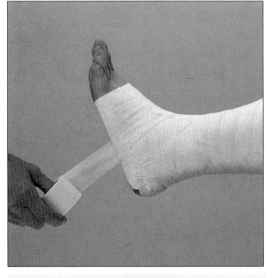

3. Pass tape under the instep heading in a posterior direction.

4. Pull the tape up and back with strong tension, moving behind the lateral malleolus (locking the heel laterally) and wrap the tape carefully around the Achilles tendon.

1. Begin taping by applying steps 1–5, 7–14 of **Ankle Rehabilitation taping, page 78.** *(Fanned stirrups may also be used if desired.)*

2. Start strip on the dorsum of the foot, crossing from lateral to medial.

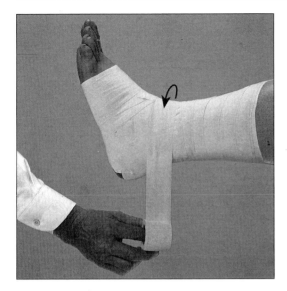

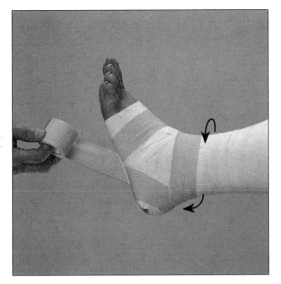

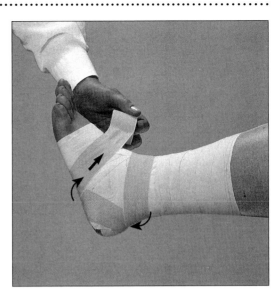

5. *Bring the tape forward on the medial side. Carefully pass over the extensor tendons anteriorly and return posteriorly.*

NOTE: Be sure to avoid wrinkling or sharp angling of the tape when crossing these tendons.

6. *Cross the Achilles tendon again bringing the tape down across the medial side of the heel, (locking it) then moving anteriorly under the plantar surface.*

NOTE: To severely limit dorsiflexion, position the ankle in more plantar flexion and pull tightly when locking the heel from each side.

7. *Pull up strongly on the lateral side and finish the strip by crossing over the starting point on the dorsum of the foot.*

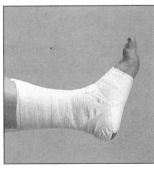

View from the medial side.

ANKLE SPRAIN REHABILITATION – ADVANCED

SUBSECTION FOR INDIVIDUAL LIGAMENT SPRAINS

The following is a detailed subsection on ankle sprains that may not be of interest to all readers. It is included to provide physiotherapists and other knowledgeable healthcare professionals intensively treating athletes with methods of specific taped support for isolated ligament sprains.

The **T.E.S.T.S.** charts in this section describe location and makeup of the individual ligaments **T**erminology. The sequence and frequency of occurrence are included with **E**tiology, **S**ymptoms, **T**reatment and **S**equelae. This section illustrates how the Rehabilitation Taping elements are adjusted and adapted for the progressive stages of healing, the anatomy of the individual ligaments, and the varying demands of different sports.

The purpose of this subsection is to show how taping can be designed to support specific ligaments and how it can be constantly progressed and adapted to meet the changing needs of the healing structure and the varying demands of different sports.

Should any given technique not provide the necessary pain-free support, consider the following:

- question the original diagnosis and reassess the injury.
- question the stage of healing: has the ankle suffered from further injury or an aggravation of the original injury thereby prolonging the sub-acute stage?
- question the appropriateness of this taping technique for this injured structure and this stage of healing.
- question your technique of application: could your skills be improved? (practice with a test strip)
- are the fundamental needs of the athlete met with adequate support yet sufficient mobility?

> NOTE: These procedures are intended as guidelines and suggestions and are by no means "carved in stone". They represent practical adaptations that have proven useful through theorization, application of knowledge, experimentation and experience.

> TIP: To develop your skills and techniques, never stop questioning, experimenting, adapting, as you apply anatomical and physiological principles to your taping.

SPECIFIC ANKLE REHABILITATION TAPING FOR: ISOLATED ANTERIOR TALO-FIBULAR LIGAMENT SPRAIN

Positioning: seated, with the calf supported and the foot held at a 90 degree angle	PROGRESSIVE STRIP ADAPTATIONS		
	SUB-ACUTE:(beginning to weightbear) • activity depends on stage of healing • how much swelling? • weightbearing only if no pain	FUNCTIONAL:(moderate to dynamic activity) • adequate support for individual ligaments • enough mobility for moderate activity	RETURN TO SPORT:(training, then competition) • reinforced support • adaptations for specific needs of sport
BASIC STRIPS			
BASIC PREPARATION: (clean, shave, spray) Prowrap anchors	• if swelling is likely, use a **felt `J`**-lateral side (bevel the edges)	• if swelling persists, continue with **felt `J`** • for increasing activity, use **heel and lace pads**	• **use heel & lace pads**
LATERAL SUPPORT: Stirrups	**modified basketweave** composed of: • **3 stirrups (vertical)** (start medially and pull up strongly on lateral side) • interlock stirrups with **2 horizontal strips** (strong lateral pull)	• continue with **modified basketweave** (extra pull on lateral side for both horizontal and vertical strips)	• continue with **modified basketweave** (extra pull particularly on lateral horizontal strips) • for more mobility, **fanned stirrups** can be used
REINFORCEMENT: Ankle locks	**lateral `V` lock** with main tension pulling up on last component (posterior vertical strip) **medial `V` lock** with main tension pulling from behind heel horizontally across medial malleolus	• continue with **I lateral V-lock** **I medial V-lock**	• continue with **lateral V-lock** **I medial V-lock**
STABILIZATION: Figure-8 variations	• **simple figure-8** (start medially and pull up strongly on lateral side) (ensure plantar flexion is restricted with this strip)	• **heel-locking figure-8** for added stability (always pull up strongly on lateral side)	• continue with **heel-locking figure-8** or • if more plantar flexion needed for sport, use **reverse figure-8** (ensure that end-range plantar flexion is limited with previous locking strips) • if tight, rigid boots are necessary, omit this step
CLOSING-UP:	• add **felt heel-lift** for weightbearing	• **heel-lift** (optional)	**Purpose:** *supports* anterior talo-fibular ligament, *prevents* inversion, *limits* inward rotation of foot, end-range eversion and end-range plantar flexion, *permits* functional plantar flexion

ANATOMICAL AREA: FOOT AND ANKLE

INJURY: ANTERIOR TALO-FIBULAR LIGAMENT SPRAIN

T ERMINOLOGY:
- anterior portion of lateral ligamentous complex
- short, superficial band of fibres
- from the anterior portion of lateral malleolus forward to the neck of the talus.
- *see* **anatomy illustration page 51, number 16.**

E TIOLOGY:
- forced inversion with plantar flexion
- "rolling over" on ankle
- the **MOST** commonly injured ankle ligament
- often secondary to inadequate rehabilitation of a previous ankle sprain (reduced proprioception).
- often injured in combination with the fibulo-calcaneal ligament.

S YMPTOMS:
- local pain, swelling and discolouration
- tenderness just anteriorly to the lateral malleollus.
- active movement testing: pain on plantar flexion with inversion
- passive movement testing: pain on plantar flexion with inversion
- resistance testing (neutral position):
  no significant pattern of pain with moderate resistance.
- stress testing
  a. pain, with or without laxity, on "anterior drawer" test (forward gliding of the talus under the tibio-fibular mortice) indicates a 1st or 2nd degree sprain
  b. instability on forward displacement of the talus away from the lateral malleolus with or without pain is indicative of a 3rd degree sprain. An audible "click" may be present.

R.I.C.E.S. : Rest, Ice, Compress, Elevate, Support

T REATMENT:
Early:
- R.I.C.E.S.
- taping, first 48 hours: **Acute Ankle injury (open basketweave) see page 72.**
- therapeutic modalities
Later:
- continued physiotherapy including:
  - therapeutic modalities
  - transverse friction massage
- modified fitness activities
- progressive pain-free rehabilitation including:
  - range of motion
  - flexibility
  - strength: non weightbearing to weightbearing (endurance, then power)
  - proprioception
- gradual painfree reintegration to sports activity with specific taping. **Ankle Rehabilitation Taping for Isolated Anterior Talo-Fibular Ligament Sprain: opposite page. (When injured in combination with fibulo-calcaneal ligament, refer to Lateral Ankle Sprain: Rehabilitation Stage taping,** *see* **page 78)**
- prevention of recurrent sprains

S EQUELAE
- anterior talo-crural instability if ligament is not supported in a shortened position during healing phase
- weakness and/or tendinitis of peroneal muscles
- chronic residual weakness of extensor digitorum longus (often injured simultaneously)
- reduced proprioception
- repeated injury caused by poor proprioception and joint instability
- chronic swelling in the sinus tarsi

SPECIFIC ANKLE REHABILITATION TAPING FOR ISOLATED CANCANEO-FIBULAR LIGAMENT SPRAIN

Positioning: seated with the calf supported and the foot held at a 90 degree angle	PROGRESSIVE STRIP ADAPTATIONS		
BASIC STRIPS	SUB ACUTE: (beginning to weightbear) • activity depends on stage of healing • how much swelling? • weightbearing only if no pain!	FUNCTIONAL: (moderate to dynamic activity) • adequate support for individual ligament • enough mobility for moderate activity	RETURN TO SPORT: (training, then competition) • reinforced support • adaptions for specific needs of sport
BASIC PREPARATION (*clean, shave, spray*) Prowrap anchors	• if swelling is likely, use a **felt 'j'**-lateral side (bevel the edges)	• if swelling persists, continue with **felt 'J'** • for increasing activity use **heel and lace pads**	• **use heel & lace pads**
LATERAL SUPPORT Stirrups	**modified basketweave** composed of: • **3 stirrups (vertical)** (start medially and pull up strongly on lateral side) • Interlock stirrups with **2 horizontal strips** (strong lateral pull)	• continue with **modified basketweave** (extra pull on lateral side, particularly for vertical strips)	• for more mobility, **fanned stirrups** can be used • if sprain is limited only to this ligament horizontal strips are now optional
REINFORCEMENT Ankle Locks	• **2 lateral locks** (pull up strongly on lateral side)	• **2 lateral locks** (extra pull on lateral side)	• continue with **2 lateral** and **1 medial** locks *or* • if tight boots are necessary, **1 lateral** lock plus **1 V-lock** replaces second lateral lock (V-lock with extra pull on horizontal part and final lateral vertical strip)
STABILIZATION Figure-8 variations	• **simple figure-8** (start medially and pull up pull up strongly on lateral side)	• **heel-locking figure-8** for added stability (always pull up strongly on lateral side)	• continue with **heel-locking figure-8** or • if more plantar flexion is needed for sport, use reverse figure-8 (ensure that end-range plantar flexion is limited with previous locking strips or with closing figure-8) • if tight, rigid boots are necessary, omit this step
CLOSING-UP:	• add **felt heel-lift** for weightbearing	• **heel-lift** optional	**Purpose:** • *supports* calcaneo-fibular ligament, • *prevents* inversion, limits end-range eversion and extreme plantar flexion, • *permits* functional plantar flexion

ANATOMICAL AREA: FOOT AND ANKLE

INJURY: CALCANEO-FIBULAR LIGAMENT SPRAIN

T ERMINOLOGY:
- middle third of the lateral ankle ligamentous complex:
- long, strong, cordlike band
- from tip of fibula inferiorly, and posteriorly to lateral tubercle on the calcaneus.
- **see anatomy illustration page 51, number 9.**

E TIOLOGY:
- a medial force on the lower leg when a dorsiflexed foot is relatively fixed in or forced into – inversion.
- more often sprained than medial side due to:
  a. a thinner, weaker less continuous ligamentous complex
  b. medial malleolus, being higher, offers less stability allowing the talus to rock medially when stressed
- most frequently injured in combination with the anterior talo-fibular ligament

S YMPTOMS:
- local pain, swelling and discolouration
- tenderness on lateral side of ankle inferior and slightly posterior to the tip of the malleolus
- active movement testing: pain on inversion
- passive movement testing: pain on inversion
- resistance testing (neutral position): no significant pattern of pain on moderate resistance
- stress testing:
  a. pain with or without some laxity on talar tilt test indicates a 1st or 2nd degree sprain
  b. instability or "opening up" on the talar tilt test (often with little or no pain) is indicative of a 3rd degree sprain of this ligament

R.I.C.E.S. : Rest, Ice, Compress, Elevate, Support

T REATMENT:
Early:
- R.I.C.E.S.
- taping: first 48 hours: **Acute Ankle Injury (open basketweave) see page 72.**
- therapeutic modalities
Later:
- continued physiotherapy including:
  - therapeutic modalities
  - transverse friction massage
  - modified fitness activities
- progressive pain-free rehabilitation including:
  - range of motion
  - flexibility
  - strength: non-weightbearing to weightbearing (endurance, then power)
  - proprioception
- gradual reintegration to sports activity with specific taped support. **See Ankle Rehabilitation Taping for Isolated Fibulo-Calcaneal Ligament Sprain: opposite page (when injured in combination with anterior talo-fibular ligament, refer to Taping for Lateral Ankle Sprain, Rehabilitation Stage: see page 78)**
- prevention of recurrence of injury

S EQUELAE:
- lateral instability if ligament is not supported in a shortened position during the healing phase
- peroneal strain often accompanies this sprain predisposing to persistent weakness and/or tendinitis of peroneal muscles
- reduced proprioception
- recurrent sprains
- chronic swelling inferior and posterior to tip of lateral malleolus
- arthritic changes

SPECIFIC ANKLE REHABILITATION TAPING FOR ISOLATED POSTERIOR TALO-FIBULAR LIGAMENT SPRAIN

Positioning: seated with the calf supported and the foot held at a 90 degree angle	PROGRESSIVE STRIP ADAPTATIONS		
	SUB ACUTE: (beginning to weightbear) • activity depends on stage of healing • how much swelling? • weightbearing only if no pain!	FUNCTIONAL: (moderate to dynamic activity) • adequate support for individual ligament • enough mobility for moderate activity	RETURN TO SPORT: (training, then competition) • reinforced support • adaptions for specific needs of sport
BASIC STRIPS			
BASIC PREPARATION (*clean, shave, spray*) Prowrap anchors	• if swelling is likely, use a **felt 'J'**-lateral side (bevel the edges)	• if swelling persists, continue with **felt 'J'** • for increasing activity use **heel and lace pads**	• **use heel & lace pads**
LATERAL SUPPORT Stirrups	**modified basketweave** composed of: • **3 stirrups (vertical)** (start medially and pull up strongly on lateral side) • Interlock stirrups with **2 horizontal strip**s (strong lateral pull)	• continue with **modified basketweave** (extra pull on lateral side, particularly for vertical strips)	• continue with **modified basketweave** (extra pull particularly on lateral horizontal strips) • for more mobility, **fanned stirrups** can be used.
REINFORCEMENT Ankle locks	• **2 lateral locks** (pull up strongly on lateral side)	• **2 lateral locks** (extra pull on lateral side) • **1 medial lock** (with less tension)	• continue with **2 lateral** and **1 medial** locks *or* • if tight boots are necessary, **1 lateral lock** plus **1 V-lock** replaces second lateral lock (V-lock with extra pull on horizontal part and final lateral vertical strip)
STABILIZATION Figure-8 variations	• **simple figure-8** (start medially and pull up pull up strongly on lateral side)	• **heel-locking figure-8** for added stability (always pull up strongly on lateral side)	• continue with **heel-locking figure-8** *or* • if injury was cause by extreme dorsiflexion or if more plantar flexion needed support, use **reverse figure-8** • if tight, rigid boots are necessary, omit this step
CLOSING-UP:	• add **felt heel-lift** for weightbearing	• continue using **heel-lift**	**Purpose:** • *supports* posterior talo-fibular ligament, • *prevents* inversion, limits dorsiflexion and lateral rotation of foot, • *permits* functional plantar flexion

Foot and Ankle

ANATOMICAL AREA: FOOT AND ANKLE

INJURY: POSTERIOR TALO-FIBULAR LIGAMENT SPRAIN

T ERMINOLOGY:
- posterior band of the lateral ligamentous complex
- deep, thick fibres
- from the posterior aspect of the malleolus to the posterior-lateral tubercle of the talus
- *see* **anatomy illustration page 51, number 11.**

E TIOLOGY:
- extreme forced dorsiflexion
- weightbearing plantar flexion with stressed external rotation of the foot
- rare as an isolated tear
- usually only ruptured in severe sprains or dislocations
- polevaulters, parachute jumpers and ice hockey players (high speed impact with boards) are prone to this injury

S YMPTOMS:
- local pain, swelling and discolouration
- tenderness posterior to the lateral malleolus deep into the peroneal tendons.
- active movement testing: pain on end-range dorsiflexion possible
- passive movement testing: posterio-lateral pain on end-range dorsiflexion
- resistance testing (neutral position): no significant pattern of pain on moderate resistance
- stress testing:
  a. posteriolateral pain often can be felt when stressing the deltoid ligament on the medial side (eversion of the calcaneus causes simultaneous pinching and compression of the injured ligament.)
  b. pain, with or without laxity on the "posterior drawer" test, backward gliding of the talus under the tibia, (worse with outward rotation of the foot) indicates a 1st or 2nd degree sprain
  c. instability (the fibula slides forward and the head of the talus moves laterally) on backward displacement of the talus, with or without pain, indicates a 3rd degree sprain

R.I.C.E.S. : Rest, Ice, Compress, Elevate, Support

T REATMENT:
Early:
- R.I.C.E.S.
- taping: first 48 hours: **Acute Ankle Injury (open basketweave)** *see* **page 72**.
- therapeutic modalities
Later:
- continued physiotherapy including:
  - therapeutic modalities
  - transverse friction massage (this ligament is difficult to access: deep in the peroneal tendons)
- modified fitness activities
- progressive pain-free rehabilitation:
  - range of motion
  - flexibility
  - strength: non-weightbearing to weightbearing (endurance, then power)
  - proprioception
- gradual pain-free reintegration to sports activity with specific taping. ***See* Ankle Rehabilitation Taping for Isolated Posterior Talo-Fibular Sprains: opposite page**.
- prevention of further sprains

S EQUELAE:
- lateral instability if ligament is not supported in a shortened position during the healing phase
- weakness of ankle musculature
- reduced proprioception
- peroneal weakness and/or tendinitis

SPECIFIC ANKLE REHABILITATION TAPING FOR: ISOLATED DELTOID LIGAMENT SPRAIN

Positioning: seated with the calf supported and the foot held at a 90 degree angle	**PROGRESSIVE STRIP ADAPTATIONS**		
	SUB ACUTE: (beginning to weightbear) • activity depends on stage of healing • how much swelling? • weightbearing only if no pain!	FUNCTIONAL: (moderate to dynamic activity) • adequate support for individual ligament • enough mobility for moderate activity	RETURN TO SPORT: (training, then competition) • reinforced support • adaptions for specific needs of sport
BASIC STRIPS			
BASIC PREPARATION (*clean, shave, spray*) Prowrap anchors	• if swelling is likely, use a **felt horseshoe**-medial side (bevel the edges)	• if swelling persists, continue with **felt horseshoe** • for increasing activity use **heel and lace pads**	• **use heel and lace pads**
LATERAL SUPPORT Stirrups	**modified basketweave** composed of: • **3 stirrups (vertical)** (start laterally and pull up strongly on medial side) • Interlock stirrups with **2 horizontal strips**	• continue with **modified basketweave** (extra pull on medial side, for both horizontal and vertical strips)	• continue with **modified basketweave** (extra pull particularly on medial side) • for more mobility, **fanned stirrups** can be used.
REINFORCEMENT Ankle locks	• **2 medial locks** (pull up strongly on lateral side)	• **2 medial locks** (extra pull on lateral side) • **1 lateral lock** (with less tension)	• if tight boots are necessary, **1 medial lock** plus **1 V-lock** replaces second medial lock (V-lock with main tension pulling up on last component posterior vertical strip) **1 lateral V-lock** replaces the lateral lock (with main tension pulling up from behind heel and across anteriorly: horizontal component)
STABILIZATION Figure-8 variations	• **simple figure-8** (start tape medial to lateral and pull up strongly on medial side)	• if anterior fibres are involved, use a **heel-locking figure-8** (with medial support) *or* • if posterior fibres are involved, use a **reverse figure-8** (with medial support) (to support medial side, start tape from medial to lateral and always pull up strongly on the medial side)	• continue with **medial heel-locking figure-8** *or* • if more plantar flexion is needed for sport, or posterior fibers are involved, use **reverse figure-8** (supporting medial side) • if tight, rigid boots are necessary, omit this step
CLOSING-UP:	• add **felt heel-lift** for weightbearing	• when posterior fibres are involved, continue to use **heel-lift**	**Purpose:** • *supports* medial collateral ligament complex; • *prevents* eversion, limits dorsiflexion and lateral • *limits* end-range inversion and extreme flexion, • *permits* functional plantar flexion

ANATOMICAL AREA: FOOT AND ANKLE

INJURY: DELTOID LIGAMENT SPRAIN

T ERMINOLOGY:
- medial lateral ligamentous complex
- superficial and deep portions
- from the medial malleolus anteriorly to the navicular (superficial) and to the talus (deep) inferiorly to the calcaneus and posteriorly to the talus (both superficial and deep fibres)
- *see* **anatomy illustration page 51, numbers 1–4.**

E TIOLOGY:
- a lateral force on the lower leg when foot is relatively fixed in extension.
- less often sprained than lateral complex due to:
- thicker, stronger, more continuous ligament fibres;
- lateral malleolus being lower offers more stability to medial side by preventing a lateral talar tilt.
- occurs in wrestlers and parachute jumpers

S YMPTOMS:
- local pain, swelling and discolouration
- locations of tenderness around medial malleolus is indicative of injury site
- active movement testing: pain on eversion
- passive movement testing: pain on eversion
- resistance testing (neutral position): no significant pattern of pain on moderate resistance
- stress testing:
  a. medial pain with or without some laxity on talar-tilt test in 1st and 2nd degree sprains
  b. anterior pain with or without some laxity on anterior drawer test is indicative of injury to the anterior fibres – 1st and 2nd degree sprains
  c. posterior pain with or without some laxity on the posterior drawer test is indicative of damage to the posterior fibres – 1st and 2nd degree sprains
  d. complete instability on any of the above three tests is indicative of a 3rd degree sprain which is often less painful than 2nd degree

R.I.C.E.S. : Rest, Ice, Compress, Elevate, Support

T REATMENT:
Early:
- R.I.C.E.S.
- taping: first 48 hours: **Acute Ankle Injury (open basketweave with medial reinforcement)** *see* **page 72**.
- therapeutic modalities
- continued physiotherapy including:
  - therapeutic modalities
  - transverse friction massage
- modified fitness activities
- progressive pain-free rehabilitation including:
  - range of motion
  - flexibility
  - strength: non-weightbearing to weightbearing (endurance, then power)
  - proprioception
- gradual pain-free reintegration to sports activity with specific taping. ***See*** **Rehabilitation Taping for Isolated Deltoid Ligament Sprains: opposite page.**
- prevention of recurrent sprains

S EQUELAE:
- medial instability if ligament is not supported in a shortened position during the healing phase
- reduced proprioception
- weakness of ankle musculature
- longer healing time
- tibialis anterior tendinitis or associated strain

Deltoid Ligament

SPECIFIC ANKLE REHABILITATION TAPING FOR: ISOLATED ANTERIOR TIBO-FIBULAR LIGAMENT SPRAIN

Positioning: seated with the calf supported and the foot held at a 10 degrees of plantar flexion	PROGRESSIVE STRIP ADAPTATIONS		
BASIC STRIPS	SUB ACUTE: (beginning to weightbear) • activity depends on stage of healing • how much swelling? • weightbearing only if no pain!	FUNCTIONAL: (moderate to dynamic activity) • adequate support for individual ligament • enough mobility for moderate activity	RETURN TO SPORT: (training, then competition) • reinforced support • adaptions for specific needs of sport
BASIC PREPARATION (*clean, shave, spray*) Prowrap anchors	• if swelling is likely, use a **felt horseshoe**-lateral side (bevel the edges)	• if swelling persists, continue with **felt horseshoe** • for increasing activity use **heel and lace pads**	• **use heel and lace pads**
LATERAL SUPPORT Stirrups	**modified basketweave** composed of: • **3 stirrups (vertical)** (start under foot and pull up equally on both sides) • Interlock stirrups with **2 horizontal strips**	• continue with **modified basketweave** (extra pull on medial side for horizontal strips)	• continue with **modified basketweave** (ensure foot is held in slight plantar flexion) • if much plantar flexion is needed for sport, **fanned stirrups** can be used
REINFORCEMENT Ankle locks	• **I lateral V-lock** (extra pull on horizontal part and final lateral vertical strip)	• **I lateral V-lock** (extra pull on horizontal part and final vertical strip) • **I medial V-lock** (extra pull on final vertical strip)	• continue as before with **I lateral V-lock** plus **I medial V-lock**
STABILIZATION Figure-8 variations	• **simple figure-8** (ensure that extreme plantar flexion is restricted with this strip)	• **reverse figure-8** (for added stability and prevention of dorsiflexion) (extra pull when crossing heel – both laterally and medially)	• continue with **reverse figure-8** (ensure that end-range plantar flexion is limited with previous locking strips or with closing figure-8) • if tight, rigid boots are necessary omit this step
CLOSING-UP:	• initially add a 1.5 cm (3.4 in.) thick **felt heel-lift** for weightbearing to avoid dorsiflexion	• **heel-lift** imperative	**Purpose:** • *supports* medial collateral ligament complex; • *prevents* eversion, limits dorsiflexion and lateral • *limits* end-range inversion and extreme flexion, • *permits* functional plantar flexion **Note:** this taping does not directly reinforce the fibres of the injured ligament, but reduces the stresses caused by extremes of motion

ANATOMICAL AREA: FOOT AND ANKLE

INJURY: ANTERIOR INFERIOR TIBIO-FIBULAR LIGAMENT SPRAIN

T ERMINOLOGY:
- anterior aspect of the ligamentous mortice of the talo-crucial joint (ankle proper) running from the anterio-lateral border of the tibia to the anterio-medial border of the fibula meeting just superior to the talus. This ligament is thinner and weaker than its counterpart, the posterior inferior tibio-fibular ligament.
- *see* **anatomy illustration page 51, number 10.**

E TIOLOGY:
- stressed in full dorsoflexion: the wider aspect of the talus jams between the malleoli
- stressed severely when a dorsoflexed foot is rotated laterally forcing the malleoli to separate
- can be accompanied by posterior fibulo calcaneal ligament sprain.
- common injury in competitive alpine skiing

S YMPTOMS:
- local pain, swelling and discolouration
- tenderness anteriorly on palpation between the tibia and fibula just superior to the talus
- active movement testing: pain on dorsiflexion at end-range; increased with active eversion
- passive movement testing: pain on dorsiflexion at end-range
- resistance testing (neutral position): no significant pattern of pain on moderate resistance
- stress testing:
  a. palpable displacement when squeezing malleoli together (may be accompanied by pain from pinching of ligament fibres)
  b. marked diastasis (opening up) of malleoli on forced varus in 3rd degree sprains
  c. in chronic cases, there is often an audible click on forced varus into an excessive range

R.I.C.E.S. : Rest, Ice, Compress, Elevate, Support

T REATMENT:
Early:
- R.I.C.E.S.
- taping: first 48 hours: Acute Ankle Injury (open basketweave) *see* **page 72**. (Position with slight plantar flexion.)
- therapeutic modalities
Later:
- continued physiotherapy including:
  - therapeutic modalities
  - transverse friction massage
- modified fitness activities
- progressive pain-free rehabilitation including:
  - range of motion
  - flexibility
  - strength: non-weightbearing to weightbearing (endurance, then power)
  - proprioception
- prevention of recurrent sprains
- gradual pain-free reintegration to sports activity with specific taping. *See* **Rehabilitation Taping for Isolated Anterior Inferior Tibio-Fibular Ligament Sprains: opposite page**.
- needs greater non-weightbearing (NWB) rehabilitation phase due to inherent displacing stress caused by weightbearing.

S EQUELAE:
- lateral talo-crural instability if ligament is not supported in shortened position during healing phase
- permanent instability of the ankle mortice
- dysfunction of the superior tibio-fibular joint
- peroneal strain and residual weakness often accompanies this sprain
- weakness of all ankle musculature
- recurrent injury

TAPING FOR CALF CONTUSION OR STRAIN

Purpose:
- applies localized specific compression to the bruised or torn tissue (prevents subsequent swelling, bleeding or muscle fibre tearing in the area)
- supports the triceps surae (calf) muscles with elastic reinforcement assisting plantar flexion
- prevents full stretch of the musculo-tendinous unit by restricting dorsiflexion
- limits inversion significantly when heel lock is used
- allows full plantar flexion and eversion

Indications for use:
- gastrocnemius or soleus (calf) strain in muscle bulk or musculo-tendinous junction
- gastrocnemius or soleus (calf) muscle bulk contusion ("Charley-horse")

MATERIALS:

razor
skin toughener spray
7.5 cm (3 in.) elastic adhesive tape
3.8 cm (1.5 in.) non-elastic white tape
10 cm (4 in.) elastic wrap
1.5 cm (2/3 in.) felt heel lift

NOTES:
- The exact site of the contusion or strain must be localized.
- Prowrap is not recommended as it significantly lessens the effectiveness of this taping technique.
- Icing of the injured muscle should start immediately.
- Flexibility starts as soon as the compression tape is applied by actively conditioning the dorsi-flexors (opposite muscle group).

For additional details regarding an injury example see TESTS chart page 114.

Positioning:

Lying prone at the end of a low bench with a folded towel placed under the thigh superior to (above) the patella (kneecap) and the calf extending over the end of the bench.

Procedure:

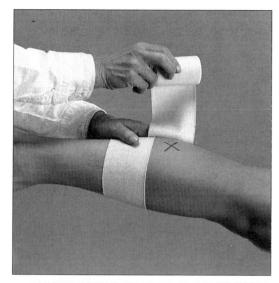

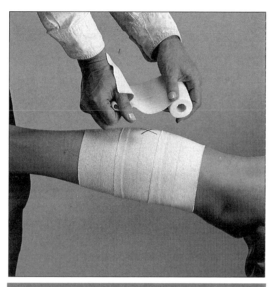

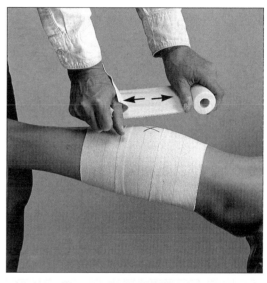

1. *Clean, shave and dry the area to be taped, checking for cuts, abrasions and sensitive skin.*

2. *Spray skin toughener or quick dry adhesive spray circumferentially to the entire calf and let dry completely.*

3. *Localize the exact site of the contusion or muscle strain. Beginning 7.5 cm (3 in.) below the lower aspect of the injury, using light tension, wrap 7.5 cm (3 in.) elastic adhesive tape around the limb. Repeat this strip overlapping the previous one by 1.5 cm. (2/3 in.) until the entire injured area is covered and surpassed by 7.5 cm (3 in.).*

NOTE: This first layer of tape forms a foundation for the compression strips which avoids excessive tension on the skin.

4a. *Prepare to apply the first pressure strip directly below the centre of the site of injury: fold back 10 cm (4 in.) at the end of a roll of 7.5 cm (3 in.) elastic adhesive tape in one hand, and hold the remainder of the roll in the other.*

4b. *Stretch the tape fully, and keep it stretched laterally.*

Calf Strain

111

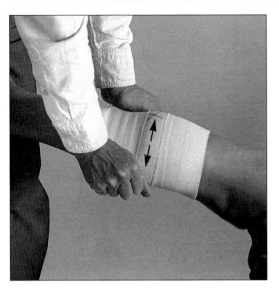

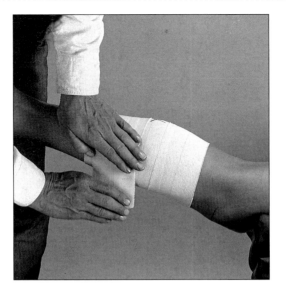

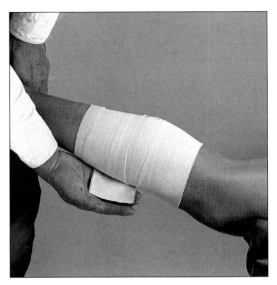

4c. *Apply strong pressure to the limb equally with both hands while maintaining the lateral stretch until the tape reaches 3/4 of the way around the limb.*

4d. *Being careful to keep the strip from detaching, release the tension while holding the stretched part against the limb, before adhering the tape end without any tension at all.*

4e. *Complete encircling the limb with the other end of the strip in the same manner, completely overlapping the tape ends at the back.*

NOTE: Application of this strip causes some discomfort.

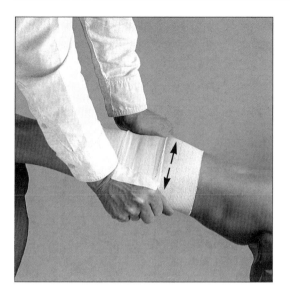

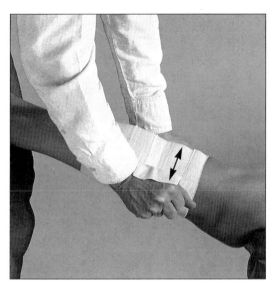

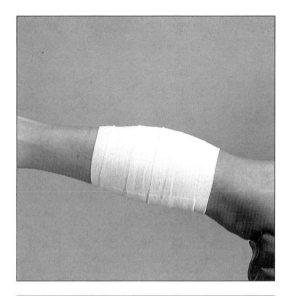

5. *Repeat the pressure strip overlapping by half the tape's width above the last strip more proximally, focusing the pressure directly over the injury.*

NOTE: This will be quite painful when pressure is applied directly to the injury site.

6. *Continue repeating the pressure strips more proximally until the entire tape base is covered.*

TIP: Ensure that the tape job extends at least one full tape-width lower and higher than the area of injury.

NOTE: The finished compression taping should have no wrinkles, should be neat in appearance and have continuous, localized pressure over the injured site from distal to proximal.

7. *For dynamic support, use the compression taping as the proximal anchor and apply the Achilles tendon taping technique. This will protect and support the entire musculo-tendinous unit for weightbearing activity.* **(see next technique page 115)**

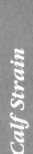

Calf Strain

ANATOMICAL AREA: FOOT AND ANKLE

INJURY: CALF STRAIN

TERMINOLOGY:
- gastrocnemius or soleus strain. **Also: Contusion; chart page 38**
- Achilles tendon complex strain: "pulled" heel cord
- degree of severity: 1st to 3rd; *see* **Strains chart see page 37**.
- torn Achilles tendon – 3rd degree strain

ETIOLOGY:
- sudden forced dorsiflexion during active plantar flexion
- explosive plantar flexion against resistance
- overstretching
- external impact to calf (contusion)
- inadequate warmup

SYMPTOMS:
- history of sudden sharp pain
- "pop" sensation
- feeling of "being shot" in the calf
- varying degrees of pain at injury site
- local swelling and gradual discolouration
- active movement testing:
  no significant pain on non-weightbearing movements
  calf pain on active plantar flexion if weightbearing
  calf pain on dorsiflexion if tight calf is being stretched
- passive movement testing:
  pain on dorsiflexion (1st and 2nd degrees)
- resistance testing (neutral position):
  a. pain on mild to moderate resistance and weakness of plantar flexion
    (1st and 2nd degrees of severity)
  b. inability to plantar flex with little or no pain is indicative of 3rd
    degree of severity (complete rupture) **See notes opposite page
    (115) for 3rd degree Strain Testing**.

TREATMENT:
Early:
- R.I.C.E.S.
- taping: **for Compression Taping see page 110**
- heel lift
- therapeutic modalities
- active contraction of dorsiflexors to induce relaxation and improve
  flexibility of calf (isometric at first)

Later:
- continued physiotherapy including:
  • therapeutic modalities
  • flexibility
  • strengthening
- proprioception
- rehabilitation program:
  non-weightbearing initially, progressing to dynamic pain-free
  reintegration with taped support **For Achilles Tendon taping** *see*
  opposite page (115).
- transverse friction massage (only after several weeks when scar tissue is
  adhering)

SEQUELAE:
- scarring
- haematoma if massaged too early
- inflexibility
- weakness
- highly prone to re-straining/cramping

R.I.C.E.S. : Rest, Ice, Compress, Elevate, Support

ANATOMICAL AREA: FOOT AND ANKLE

TAPING FOR ACHILLES TENDON INJURY

Purpose
- supports the Achilles tendon with elastic reinforcement assisting plantar flexion
- prevents full stretch of the musculo-tendinous unit by restricting full dorsoflexion
- limits inversion significantly when heel lock is used
- permits full plantar flexion and eversion

Indications for use:
- Achilles tendon strain
- Achilles tendinitis
- diffuse heel pain (possible bursitis)
- calf strain; use in combination with **Compression Taping, page 110**.
- calf contusion; use in combination with **Compression Taping, page 110**.
- peroneus longus strain or tendinitis: use in combination with **Peroneus Longus Support Strips page 122**.
- tibialis posterior strain or tendinitis; use in combination with **Tibialis Posterior Support Strips page 126**.

MATERIALS:

razor
skin toughener spray
prowrap
3.8 cm (1.5 in.) white tape
5 cm (2 in.) elastic adhesive tape
7.5 cm (3 in.) elastic adhesive tape
2 cm (3/4 in.) felt or dense foam heel lift

NOTES:
- Be sure that a thorough assessment has been done.
  In third degree strains (complete rupture):
  a. passive squeezing of the calf in a prone position will not produce plantar flexion of the foot on the injured side. (Positive Thompson Test).
  b. a palpable gap may be present.
  c. a passive dorsiflexion will be significantly freer on the injured side and does not cause extreme pain.
IF A THIRD DEGREE STRAIN IS SUSPECTED, THE ATHLETE MUST BE SEEN BY AN ORTHOPAEDIC SURGEON AS EARLY AS POSSIBLE.
- Evaluate the site of injury, pain may be located at the base of the Achilles tendon, in the belly of the calf muscle, or at the musculo-tendinous junction.
- During taping, neutral alignment of the foot can be controlled by the taper whose thigh is used as counter-pressure against the athlete's great toe.
- Because Achilles taping pulls the foot into plantar flexion, the ankle is rendered less stable and the risk of an inversion sprain is increased. (Step 13 demonstrates preventative measures.)
- Once taped, a felt or foam heel-lift in the athlete's shoe will shorten and help support the Achilles tendon by improving its mechanical advantage.

For additional details regarding an injury example see TESTS chart page 121.

Positioning:

Lying prone (face down) with the shin resting on a cushioned support and the foot protruding over the edge of the table. [For steps 1-4 it is more convenient to have the subject supine (face up) with the lower limb extending over the end of the table at mid-calf.]

Procedure:

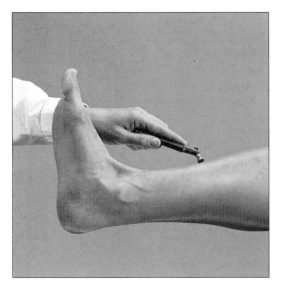

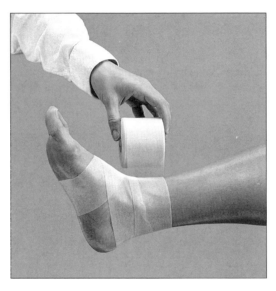

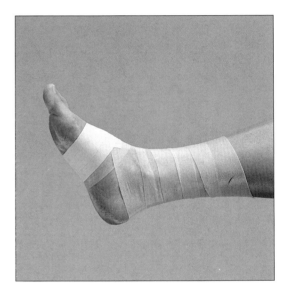

1. *Clean, shave and dry the area, checking for skin irritations, cuts or abrasions.*
2. *Spray with skin toughener or quick dry adhesive.*

3. *Apply prowrap without tension around ankle up to lower 1/3 of calf.* ***AVOID WRINKLING****.*

NOTE: Heel and lace pads should be used when taping is to enable athlete to resume playing.

4. *Apply two circumferential anchors of 3.8 cm (1.5 in.) white tape at the level of heads of metatarsals.*

TIP: Be sure to allow for some splaying of the metatarsals.

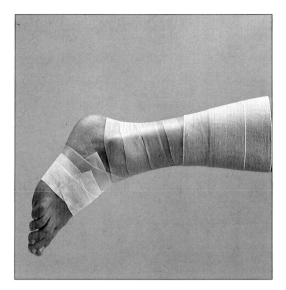

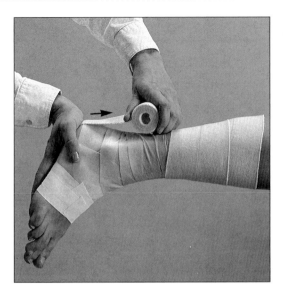

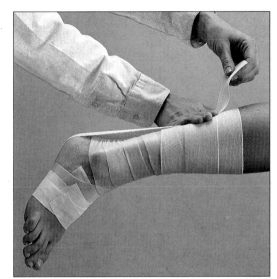

5. *Have the athlete turn to lie prone (face down) to facilitate the rest of the taping technique. Using only slight tension, apply two circumferential anchors of 5 cm (2 in.) elastic adhesive tape at mid-belly of calf muscle.*

6. *Apply the first vertical strip using 7.5 cm (3 in.) adhesive elastic tape:*

a. *Fix it firmly, **without tension**, to the plantar surface of foot.*

b. *Pull upwards, from the centre of the back of the calcaneus (heel), **with strong tension**, to lower edge of calf anchor.*

> TIP: Allow the ankle to plantar flex.

6c. *Support this strip without loosening its tension and carefully apply the last 5 cm (2 in.) of tape with virtually **no tension**, before cutting the tape from the roll.*

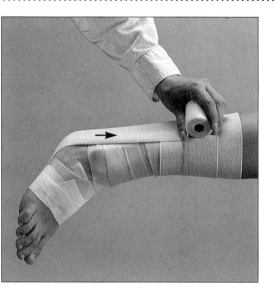

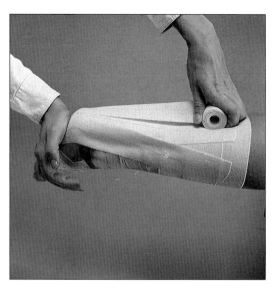

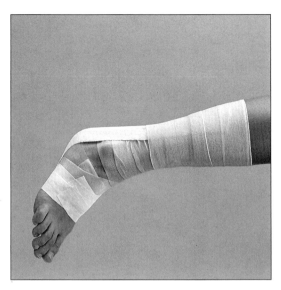

7. *Repeat step 6, passing just laterally to the centre of back of heel, pulling up firmly to control the medial tilt of the calcaneus.*

TIP: Maintain strong tension while adhering the upper end of this strip to the calf anchor before cutting the tape.

8. *Repeat step 6, passing just medially to centre of back of heel, controlling the lateral tilt and forming a "V" over the Achilles tendon posteriorly before reanchoring strips at both ends.*

NOTE: Special reinforcement strips should be added after this strip before going on to step 9. See page 122 for Peroneus Longus Adaptation and page 126 for Tibialis Posterior Adaptation.

9. *Close up calf portion of the tape job with circumferential strips of elastic adhesive tape.*

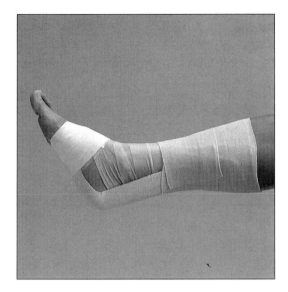

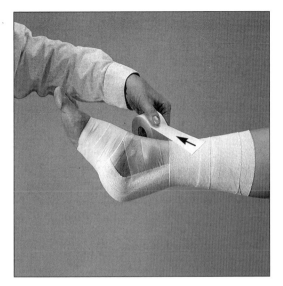

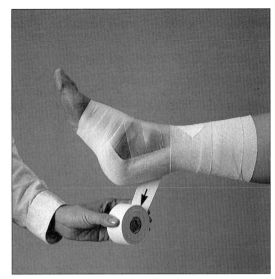

10. Reposition the athlete in a supine (lying face up) position to facilitate the next steps.
11. Apply a white tape anchor to the mid-foot, over heads of the metatarsals (forefoot).
12. Close up foot portion of the tape job with circumferential strips of white tape, overlapping each previous strip by 1/2.

13. A lateral ankle lock is appled to offer stability:
   a. Beginning on the medial side of the upper anchor, pass down across the anterior shin.

NOTE: Once the foot is held in plantar flexion, ankle stability is compromised based on the demands of the sport and the individual's ankle stability; the use of one or two ankle locks is recommended as outlined in the following optional procedure. (Steps 13 and 14)

13b. Wind the tape around behind the Achilles tendon, to catch the heel from the medial side.

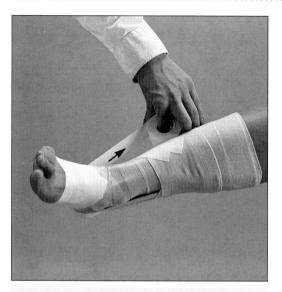

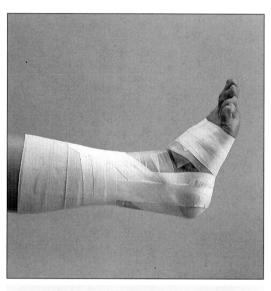

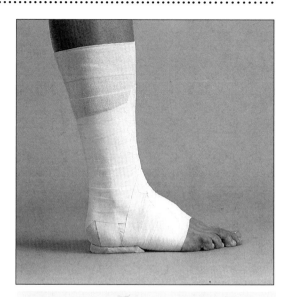

13c. *Lock the heel and pull the tape up with strong tension on the lateral side before affixing it to the upper anchors.*

14. *Repeat step 13 (a–c) a second time on the lateral side.*
15. *Reanchor these locks.*

NOTE: A medial lock can also be applied to reinforce stability in particularly vulnerable ankles.

16. *Close up the entire tape job, covering any open areas.*

17. *Test limits of taping restriction to ensure adequate pain-free support.*
    a. *Dorsiflexion must be limited by at least 30°*
    b. *There should be no pain on passive dorsiflexion.*

18. *For the acute and sub acute stages cut a 2 cm (3/4 in.) felt heel lift, bevelled at the anterior (front) edge, and place it under the heel to raise it thereby reducing tension on the tendon.*

TIP: it is best to add heel lifts to both feet for a balanced gait.

INJURY: ACHILLES TENDINITIS

T ERMINOLOGY:
- Achilles tendon inflammation (irritation)
- chronic heel cord strain

E TIOLOGY:
- structural strain from repeated quick push-offs as in repetitive running
- sudden change in training; increased distance, speed or intensity; change of terrain (example: hills vs. level ground)
- new footwear – inadequate heel support
- inadequate warmup and stretching
- subsequent to a gastrocnemius (calf) strain

S YMPTOMS:
- tenderness plus swelling around tendon
- localized pain (usually mid-tendon) spreads as condition progresses
- acute posterior heel pain on weightbearing plantar flexion (particularly after resting)
- active motion testing: possible pain on plantar flexion
- passive movement testing: usually painful on dorsiflexion
- resistance testing (neutral position): possible weakness and marked pain on moderate resistance

T REATMENT:
- physiotherapy including:
  - ice
  - therapeutic modalities
  - transverse friction massage
- **Achilles Tendon taping, page 115**.
- heel lift
- modified training program
- total rehabilitation program with emphasis on full flexibility, eccentric strengthening through range of motion and dynamic proprioception
- progressive reintegration to regular sports activity with taped support as above

S EQUELAE:
- persistent pain
- scarring/thickening of tendon
- inflexibility
- weakness of calf
- imbalance of ankle musculature flexibility and/or strength
- bursitis
- calcification of tendon or bursa

Achilles Tendinitis

ANATOMICAL AREA: FOOT AND ANKLE

TAPING FOR: PERONEUS LONGUS TENDON INJURY

Purpose:
- supports peroneus longus tendon with elastic reinforcement assisting plantar flexion with eversion
- prevents full stretch of the musculo-tendinous unit by restricting dorsiflexion and inversion
- permits full plantar flexion plus eversion

Indications for use:
- peroneus longus tendon strain
- peroneus longus tendinitis

MATERIALS:

razor
skin toughener spray
prowrap
5 cm (2 in.) elastic adhesive tape
7.5 cm (3 in.) elastic adhesive tape
2 cm (3/4 in.) felt or dense foam heel lift
3.8 cm (1.5 in.) white tape

NOTES:
- Ensure that a thorough assessment has been done.
- In 3rd degree strains (complete rupture);
  a. there is no isolated strength of eversion with plantar flexion
  b. there is no significant pain on passive inversion with dorsiflexion
- If a 3rd degree strain is suspected, a sports medicine specialist should be consulted as soon as possible to evaluate indications for surgery depending on age, fitness level, and demands of the sport.

For additional details regarding an injury example see TESTS chart page 125.

Positioning:

Lying supine (face up) then prone (face down) with the shin resting on a cushioned support and the foot protruding over the edge of the table.

Procedure:

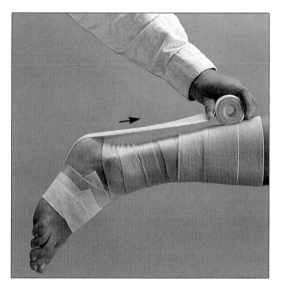

1. *Begin taping by applying steps 1–8 of* **Achilles tendon taping, page 115**.

NOTE: Strips must be reanchored before proceeding.

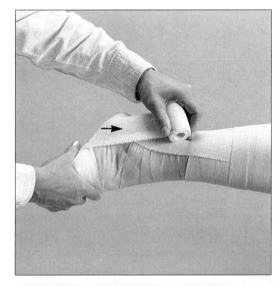

2a. *Affix, without tension, a strip of 5 cm (2 in.) elastic adhesive tape to the plantar surface of the foot starting on the medial side leading diagonally across to the lateral side of the heel.*

b. *Holding the foot in plantar flexion and significant eversion, pull the tape up strongly across the lateral side of the heel.*

TIP: following the direct line of pull of this tendon.

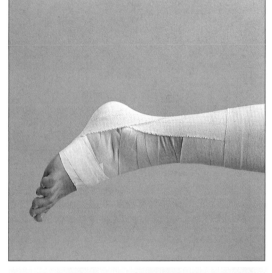

2c. *Maintain strong tension and affix the tape to the calf anchors.*

TIP: Apply the last 5 cm (2 in.) of tape with no tension before cutting tape from roll.

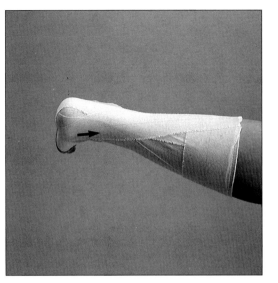

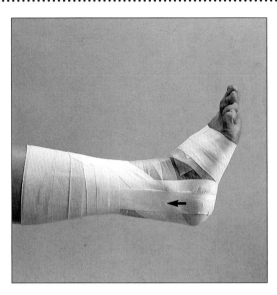

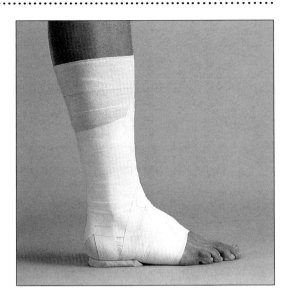

3. *Repeat strip **2a–2c** a second time, slightly more anterior (1 cm, 1/2").*

4. *Continue the tape job with the **Achilles taping technique, step 9 page 118** (lateral heel-locking reinforcement is less critical in this tape job because the ankle is already pulled into eversion).*

5. *Test limits of taping restriction to ensure adequate pain-free support:*
   a. *Dorsiflexion with inversion must be restricted by at least 30°*
   b. *There should be no pain on passive dorsiflexion with inversion.*

TIP: Use a heel lift to reduce the strain on the tendon when weightbearing.

ANATOMICAL AREA: FOOT AND ANKLE

INJURY: PERONEUS LONGUS TENDINITIS

T ERMINOLOGY:
- chronic overuse syndrome of peroneus longus
- tenosynovitis (inflammation of tendon and sheath)

E TIOLOGY:
- poor foot biomechanics (more common with high arches)
- weakness and/or inflexibility of lateral ankle muscles
- chronic overstretch or overuse
- subsequent to peroneus longus strain or chronic ankle sprains
- inadequate foot support
- repeated running on hard surfaces
- sudden change in terrain, speed, intensity, frequency, resistance, etc.
- uncommon incidence: seen in figure skaters

S YMPTOMS:
- swelling and cramping
- localized thickening and tenderness of tendon
- localized heat and redness along tendon possible
- crepitation
- active movement testing:
  weightbearing: pain on plantar flexion particularly if associated with eversion
  non-weightbearing : possible pain on plantar flexion with eversion
  localized pain during active dorsiflexion with inversion (if tight) peroneus is being stretched
- passive movement testing:
  pain on dorsiflexion with inversion (1st and 2nd degree Sprains)
- resistance testing (neutral position):
  pain with or without weakness on eversion with plantar flexion

> **NOTE:** Inability to evert in plantar flexion with little or no pain indicative of a 3rd degree strain – tendon rupture. See page 37 for 3rd degree strains.

T REATMENT:
- physiotherapy including:
  - ice
  - therapeutic modalities (laser or ultrasound particularly helpful)
  - transverse friction massage
- modified activity initially
- taping **for Peroneus Longus adaption of Achilles Tendon Taping see page 122**
- selective strengthening of Peroneus Longus; NWB (non-weightbearing) initially, progressing gradually to eccentric FWB (full weightbearing)
- flexibility then strengthening of all ankle musculature
- thorough biomechanical assessment and re-education
- orthotics may be indicated
- gradual (pain-free) reintegration to sports activities with taped support as above
- total rehabilitation: progressive exercise program for flexibility, strength and dynamic proprioception

S EQUELAE:
- scarring
- inflexibility
- weakness of evertors
- muscle imbalance
- chronic tendinitis
- chronic subluxing or dislocating tendons
- predisposition to ankle sprains
- lateral compartment syndrome

Peroneus Longus Strain

ANATOMICAL AREA: FOOT AND ANKLE

TAPING FOR: TIBIALIS POSTERIOR TENDON INJURY

Purpose:

- supports tibialis posterior tendon with elastic reinforcement assisting plantar flexion with inversion
- prevents full stretch of the musculo-tendinous unit by restricting dorsiflexion and eversion
- limits inversion significantly when heel lock is used
- permits full plantar flexion

Indications for use:

- tibialis posterior tendon strain
- tibialis posterior tendinitis

MATERIALS:

razor
skin toughener spray
prowrap
5 cm (2 in.) elastic adhesive tape
7.5 cm (3 in.) elastic adhesive tape
2 cm (3/4 in.) felt or dense foam heel lift
3.8 cm (1.5 in.) white tape

NOTES:
- Ensure that a thorough assessment has been done.
- In 3rd degree strain (complete rupture);
  a. there is no isolated strength of inversion with plantar flexion
  b. there is no significant pain on passive eversion with dorsiflexion
- If a 3rd degree strain is suspected, a sports medicine specialist should be consulted as soon as possible to evaluate indications for surgery depending on age, fitness level, and demands of the sport.

For additional details regarding an injury example see TESTS chart page 129.

Positioning:

Lying supine (face up) to begin with, then lying prone (face down) with the shin resting on a cushioned support and the foot protruding over the edge of the table.

Procedures:

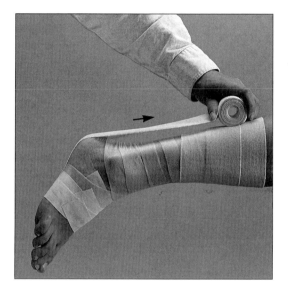

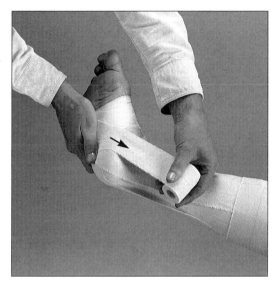

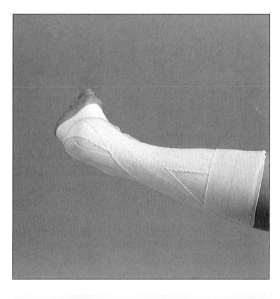

1. Begin taping by applying steps 1–8 of **Achilles tendon taping, page 115.**

NOTE: Reanchor strips before proceeding.

2a. Affix, without tension, a strip of 5 cm (2 in.) elastic adhesive tape to the plantar surface of the foot starting on the lateral side leading diagonally across to the medial side of the heel.

b. Holding the foot in plantar flexion and significant inversion, pull the tape up strongly across the medial side of the heel.

TIP: following the direct line of pull of the posterior tibialis tendon.

2c. Maintain strong tension and affix the tape to the calf anchors.

TIP: Apply the last 5 cm (2 in.) of tape with no tension before cutting

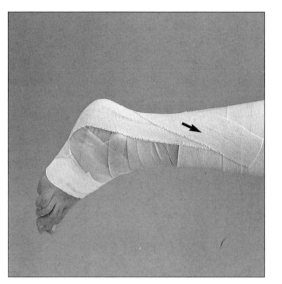

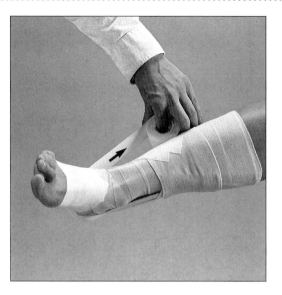

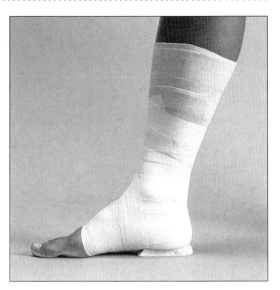

3. *Repeat strip* ***2a–2c*** *a second time, slightly more anterior (1 cm, 1/2").*

4. *Continue the tape job with the* ***Achilles taping, step 9, page 118***

NOTE: It is essential to reinforce lateral ligament structures with a heel lock to prevent inversion sprains.

5. *Test limits of taping restriction to ensure adequate pain-free support:*
   a. *Dorsiflexion with eversion must be limited by at least 30° or more*
   b. *There should be no pain on passive dorsiflexion with eversion.*

TIP: Use a heel lift to reduce the strain on the tendon when weightbearing.

ANATOMICAL AREA: FOOT AND ANKLE

INJURY: TIBIALIS POSTERIOR TENDINITIS

T ERMINOLOGY:
- chronic overuse syndrome of tibialis posterior
- shin splints
- tenosynovitis (inflammation of tendon and sheath)

E TIOLOGY:
- overly pronated or flat feet
- poor foot biomechanics (a fixed forefoot inversion with a valgus calcaneus)
- weakness and/or inflexibility of medial ankle muscles
- chronic overstretch or overuse
- subsequent to tibialis posterior strain or chronic ankle sprains
- inadequate foot support
- repeated running on hard surfaces
- sudden change in terrain, speed, intensity, frequency, resistance, etc.
- common in joggers and ballet dancers

S YMPTOMS:
- pain posterior to medial malleolus extending up to posterio-medial border of tibia (can radiate down to the medial arch).
- localized swelling and thickening of tendon
- exquisitely tender on palpation of inflamed site
- local heat and redness over tendon possible
- crepitation
- active movement testing:
  weightbearing: pain, particularly at push-off
  non-weightbearing : possible pain on plantar flexion with inversion
  pain on dorsiflexion with eversion
- passive movement testing: pain on dorsiflexion with eversion
- resistance testing (neutral position): pain with or without weakness on resisted inversion with plantar flexion

> **NOTE:** Inability to invert in plantar flexion with little or no pain indicative of a 3rd degree strain – tendon rupture. See page 37 for 3rd degree Strains.

T REATMENT:
- physiotherapy including:
  - ice
  - therapeutic modalities (laser or ultrasound particularly helpful)
  - transverse friction massage
- modified activity initially
- taping **for Tibialis Posterior adaption of Achilles Tendon Taping see page 126**
- selective strengthening of Tibialis Posterior; NWB (non-weightbearing) initially, progressing to eccentric FWB (full weightbearing)
- strengthening and flexibility of all ankle musculature
- thorough biomechanical assessment and re-education
- orthotics may be indicated
- gradual pain-free reintegration program with taped support as above
- total rehabilitation: progressive exercise program for flexibility, strength and dynamic proprioception

S EQUELAE:
- scarring
- inflexibility
- weakness of invertors
- muscle imbalance
- chronic tendinitis
- chronic shin splints
- deep posterior compartment syndrome (surgical splitting of fascia sometimes necessary in severe cases
- predisposition to stress fractures

Tibialis Posterior Strain

Chapter Seven ....

KNEE AND THIGH

The knee is a hinged weightbearing joint dependent on several structures for stability:
- **medial and lateral collateral ligaments** prevent lateral (sideways) movements
- **anterior and posterior cruciate ligaments** located centrally, prevent anterior (forward) and posterior (backward) displacement during movement.
- **two wedge-shaped menisci (cartilages)** form mechanical spacers to cushion forces, guide movements and add to total stability.

The **patella (knee-cap),** while improving the biomechanical efficiency of the quadriceps, is often the source of incapacitating knee pain.

The knee is frequently injured - especially in contact sports - due to several factors:
- heavy weightbearing demands on the knee in sports activities
- a relatively weaker medial collateral ligament with its attachments to the medial meniscus
- vulnerability of the anterior cruciate ligament.

Correct taping and treatment for knee sprains permits the athlete to continue sports participation with minimal risk of sustaining further injury. Taped support gives stability to the injured structure, enhances end-range proprioceptive feedback, and promotes healing through dynamic function.

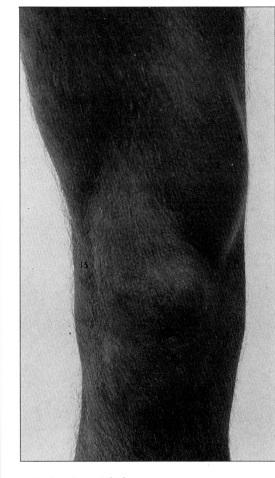

Anterior view, right knee

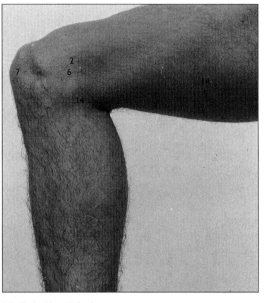

Medial side, right knee

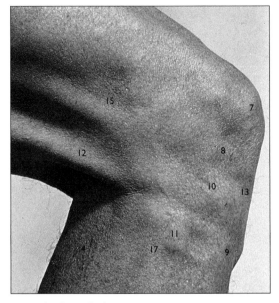

Lateral side, right knee

Behind the knee on the lateral side the rounded tendon of biceps (12) can be felt easily, with the broad strap-like iliotibial tract (15) in front of it, with a furrow between them. On the medial side two tendons can be felt—the narrow rounded semitendinosus (14) just behind the broader semimembranosus (5). At the front the patellar ligament (13) keeps the patella (7) at a constant distance from the tibial tuberosity (9), while at the side the adjacent margin of the femoral and tibial condyles can be palpated.

MUSCLES	**TENDONS**
1 QUADRICEPS: RECTUS FEMORIS	12 BICEPS FEMORIS
2 QUADRICEPS: VASTUS MEDIALIS	13 PATELLAR 'LIGAMENT'
3 QUADRICEPS: VASTUS LATERALIS	14 SEMITENDINOSIS
4 GASTROCNEMIUS	**FASCIA**
5 SEMIMEMBRANOSIS	15 ILIOTIBIAL TRACT
6 ADDUCTOR MAGNUS	**HOLLOWS**
BONES	16 POPLITEAL FOSSA OF KNEE JOINT
7 PATELLA	**NERVES**
8 MARGIN OF CONDYLE OF FEMUR	17 COMMON PERINEAL
9 TUBEROSITY OF TIBIA	
10 MARGIN OF CONDYLE OF TIBIA	
11 HEAD OF FIBULA	

TAPING FOR MEDIAL COLLATERAL LIGAMENT (MCL) KNEE SPRAIN

Purpose:
- supports the medial collateral ligament (MCL) by tightening the medial aspect of the joint line.
- prevents the last 15° of knee extension and external rotation of the tibia under the femur.
- allows almost full flexion and functional extension of the knee.

Indications for use:
- medial collateral ligament (MCL) sprains: 1st & 2nd degree
- post immobilization of 3rd degree MCL sprains
- * for medial meniscus injuries: emphasize spiral strips which cause internal rotation of the tibia

MATERIALS:

razor
skin toughener spray
prowrap
7.5 cm (3 in.) and 10 cm (4 in.) elastic adhesive tape
5 cm (2 in.) and 3.8 (1.5 in.) non-elastic white tape
15.2 cm (6 in.) elastic wrap
skin lubricant
heel and lace pads

NOTES:
To determine the degree of injury, be certain that a competent sports medicine specialist examines the athlete.
  a. medial stability should be tested at 30° of knee flexion as well as at 0°
  b. if the knee is also unstable at 0° of extension, a serious injury is suspected
  c. X-rays should be taken to rule out an avulsion fracture.
- Always assess which knee and which side of that knee was injured (the athlete may have sustained spraining on the medial aspect of the same knee and bruising on the lateral aspect).
- During exercise, increased blood circulation causes swelling of thigh muscles. Ensure that circumferential strips are affixed with only light tension, avoiding constriction and possible cramping of thigh and calf muscles.
- Avoid taping over the patella, as this can cause compression, pain, and subsequent problems.

For additional details regarding an injury example see TESTS chart page 141.

Positioning:

Standing on a stool or a chair with a roll of tape under the heel (injured side) with the knee bent slightly. The foot is turned inwards to medially rotate the tibia under the femur. (This takes the tension off the medial collateral ligament). 80% of body weight should be supported by the uninjured side.

Procedure:

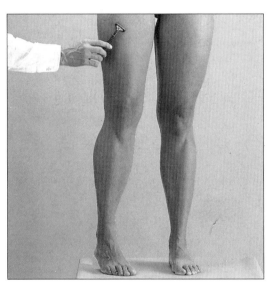

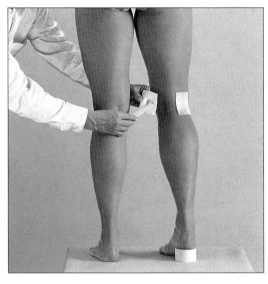

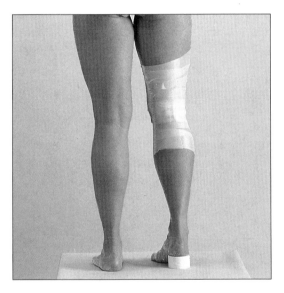

1. Clean, shave and dry the area to be taped, checking for cuts, abrasions or sensitive areas.

2. Place lubricated pads over the hamstring tendons.

3. Spray mid-thigh and mid-calf circumferentially with skin toughener or quick dry adhesive.

4. Apply prowrap from mid-calf to mid-thigh.

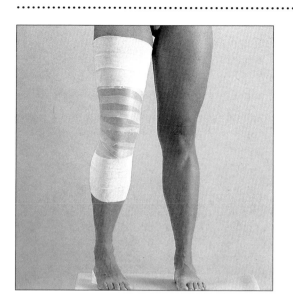

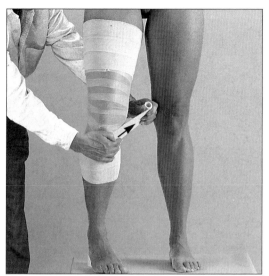

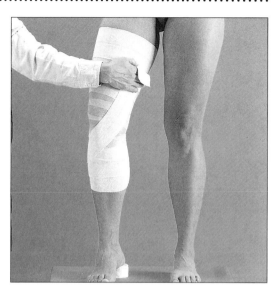

5. *Apply 2 circumferential anchors of 10 cm (4 in.) elastic adhesive tape using only slight tension, to the mid-thigh and mid-calf regions covering the skin well beyond the edge of the prowrap.*

NOTE: Re-check the athlete's position.

6. *Place a strip of 7.5 cm (3 in.) elastic adhesive tape starting from the posterio-medial aspect of the distal anchor, spiralling around the lateral side of the tibia, anteriorly. Cross medially below the patella with moderate tension, and pull proximally with strong tension over the medial joint line to the proximal anchor.*

NOTE: This strip helps to medially rotate the tibia as well as approximate the medial joint.

TIP: The last 7.5 cm (3 in.) of the strip must be applied directly to the anchor strip, and must not be applied under tension. (The tape end will peel back if tension has not been released.)

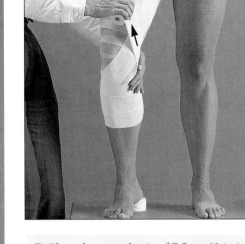

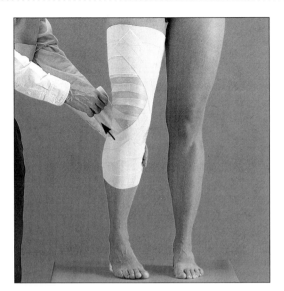

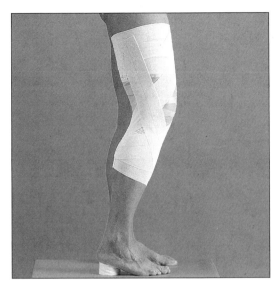

7. *Place the second strip of 7.5 cm (3 in.) elastic adhesive tape also starting from the posterio-medial aspect of the distal anchor, this time heading anteriorly on the medial side. Pull proximally with strong tension over the medial joint line to the proximal anchor anteriorly, releasing the tension only when adhering the end of the strip.*

8a. *Begin a lateral X with a strip of 7.5 cm (3 in.) elastic adhesive tape from the posterio-medial aspect of the lower leg, winding behind the tibia, (reinforcing internal rotation of the tibia) with some tension upwards on the lateral aspect of the knee above the patella to the proximal anchor anteriorly.*

8b. *Place the next strip of 7.5 cm (3 in.) elastic adhesive tape from the anterio-lateral aspect of the distal anchor, pulling proximally with some tension over the lateral joint line, to the proximal anchor.*

NOTE: These two strips form an X directly on the medial joint line, over the site of the medial collateral ligament.

NOTE: These last two strips form an X directly on the lateral joint line, with less tension. The ends interlock with the medial X over the anchors, reinforcing stability.

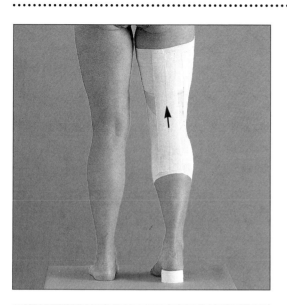

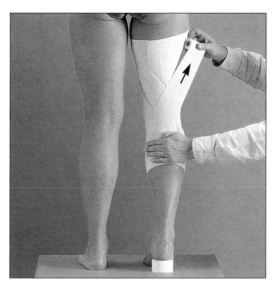

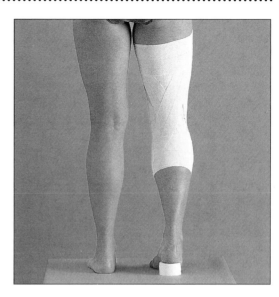

9. *With the knee still flexed, apply a vertical strip of 7.5 cm (3 in.) elastic adhesive tape from the centre of the posterior of the distal anchor to the centre of the proximal anchor to prevent hyperextension.*

TIP: Flex the knee at least 30° and use strong tension when applying this strip.

10. *Apply an X of 7.5 cm (3 in.) fully stretched elastic adhesive tape on the posterior knee.*

11. *Reanchor the tape with proximal and distal anchors .*

NOTE: This completed butterfly must be tight enough to limit the last 10–15° of knee extension.

Knee Sprain (MCL)

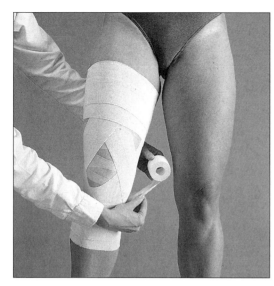

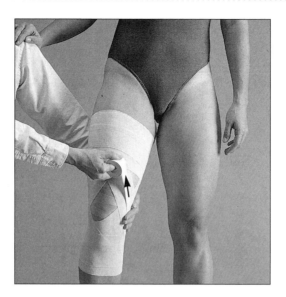

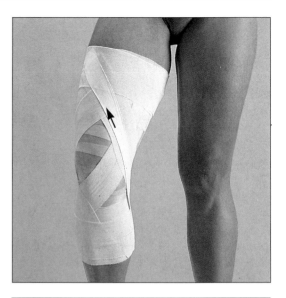

12. *Apply an oblique vertical strip of 5 cm (2 inch) white non-elastic tape from the posterior medial aspect of the lower anchor to the anterio-medial aspect of the upper anchor.*

TIP: Fold the edges of the tape back to reinforce it's strength making the portion crossing the ligament virtually unrippable.

TIP: When applying this strip, hold the distal end firmly against lower anchor while pressing the knees into extreme varus, and pull up with maximal force.

NOTE: The athlete will need to hold onto the taper's shoulder or use a nearby wall for stability at this stage.

NOTE: THE KNEE MUST REMAIN RELAXED, while the athlete's weight is borne mainly on the uninjured leg.

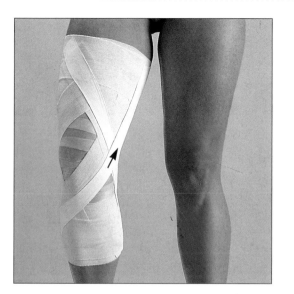

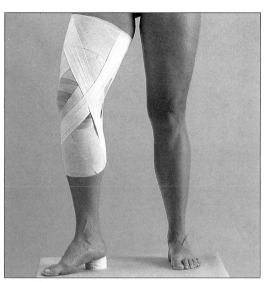

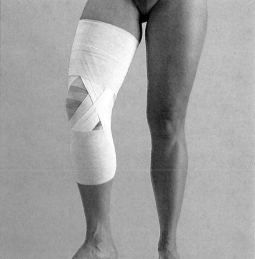

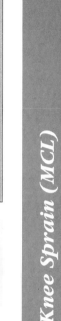

13. *Apply a second oblique vertical strip of 5 cm (2 in.) white non-elastic tape, this time from the anterior aspect of the lower anchor to the posterio-medial aspect of the upper anchor, using the same principles as outlined for step 12.*

a. *Pinch the tape edges for increased tape strength.*

b. *Apply this tape strip using maximal force upwards while pressing the knee into extreme varus.*

> NOTE: The X formed by these two strips must lie on the medial joint line, over the site of the medial collateral ligament.

14. *Repeat the white tape X, overlapping slightly anteriorly to the first white tape X.*

15. *Using light tension, re-anchor the tape job with 2 circumferential strips of 10 cm (4 in.) elastic adhesive tape over the mid-thigh anchor and 2 strips over the mid-calf anchor.*

Knee Sprain (MCL)

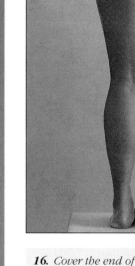

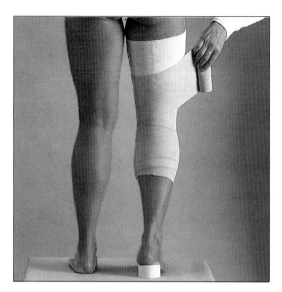

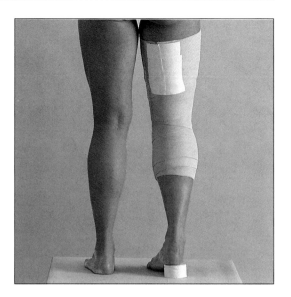

16. Cover the end of the elastic tape with two short strips of white tape to keep the elastic tape securely in place.

17. Test the degree of restriction:

a. extension must be limited by 10°

b. there must be no medial laxity

c. there must be no pain on medial stress testing inward bending of the knee, external rotation of the tibia under the femur and extension.

18. Wrap the entire tape job with an elastic wrap prior to allowing the athlete to resume activity. This gives the adhesive tape the time and heat necessary to set.

19. Tape the elastic wrap in place with white adhesive tape.

NOTES:
• For acute sprains: leave elastic wrap on for at least the first 48 hours.
• For back to sport taping leave elastic wrap on for at least 15 minutes and remove for full activity.

ANATOMICAL AREA: KNEE AND THIGH

INJURY: KNEE SPRAIN MEDIAL COLLATERAL LIGAMENT (MCL)

TERMINOLOGY
- medial collateral ligament sprain: 1st–3rd degree of severity. **(See Sprains Chart, page 36)**
- internal collateral ligament sprain: 1st–3rd degree of severity
- pulled knee

E TIOLOGY:
- excessive inward pressure forcing the knee medially into valgus (inwardly bent "knock-kneed" position). Example: a football player tackled at the knees from the left side may sustain a medial sprain of the left knee and potentially a lateral sprain of the right knee
- sudden impact forcing body laterally on a fixed foot
- often associated with other injured structures (medial meniscus, anterior cruciate: "the unhappy triad")

S YMPTOMS:
- local pain and tenderness on the medial side (inside) of the knee
- swelling , possible bruising
- active movement testing: medial pain on end-range extension
- resistance testing (neutral position): no pain on moderate resistance
- stress testing:
  a. 1st and 2nd degree sprain: medial pain with or without instability when tested at 30° knee flexion
  b. 3rd degree of severity: complete ligament rupture ("opens up"); at 30° can be less pain than with 2nd degree
  c. instability at 0° extension is indicative of a severe injury with posterior capsule involvement

T REATMENT:
Early:
- R.I.C.E.S.
- Taping: **MCL sprain page 133** (plus elastic wrap for first 48 hours)
- therapeutic modalities

NOTE: Surgery may be indicated for 3rd degree of severity.

Later:
- continued physiotherapy including:
  - therapeutic modalities
  - transverse friction massage
  - mobilizations if stiff following immobilization
  - flexibility exercises for quadriceps, hamstrings and gastrocnemeii
- strengthening exercises (isometric at first) for quadriceps and hamstrings
- gradual reintegration program with pain free taped support: **for MCL sprain,** *see* **page 133**
- total rehabilitation program for range of motion, flexibility, strength, and proprioception
- bracing may be recommended for return to activity or for continued athletic performance if chronically unstable

S EQUELAE:
- medial (valgus) laxity
- chronic instability
- weakness of quadriceps
- degeneration of medial meniscus
- osteoarthritic changes

R.I.C.E.S: Rest, Ice, Compress, Elevate, Support

Knee Sprain (MCL)

TAPING FOR LATERAL COLLATERAL LIGAMENT (LCL) SPRAINS OF THE KNEE

Purpose:
- supports the lateral collateral ligament (LCL) by tightening the lateral aspect of the joint line.
- prevents the last 15° of knee extension and restricts end range flexion slightly.
- allows functional flexion and extension of the knee.

Indications for use:
- lateral collateral ligament sprains: 1st and 2nd degree.
- post immobilization of 3rd degree LCL sprains.
- posterior cruciate ligament sprains.
- can be combined effectively with taping techniques MCL and/or ACL above for multiple knee ligament injuries.
- posterio-lateral capsular injuries (combined with ACL taping) **(see page 148)**

MATERIALS:

razor
skin toughener spray
prowrap
lubricant
heel and lace pads
10 cm (4 in.) elastic adhesive tape
7.5 cm (3 in.) elastic adhesive tape
5 cm (2 in.) non-elastic white tape
15.2 cm (6 in.) elastic wrap

NOTES:
To determine degree of injury, be certain that a competent sports medicine specialist examines the athlete
  a. lateral stability should be tested at 30° knee flexion and at 0°
  b. if the knee is also unstable medially at 0° extension, a serious injury is suspected.
  c. X-rays should be taken.
- Be certain to check both medial and lateral sides of both knees for damage resulting from lateral impact.
- Watch for peroneal nerve damage, weakness of eversion (outward pushing) of foot and decreased sensation – lateral side of injured leg.
- Keep tabs on any necessary medical follow-up.
- Ensure that anchor tightness does not compromise circulation.

For additional details regarding an injury example see TESTS chart page 146..

Positioning:

Standing on a stool or a chair with a roll of tape under the heel (injured side) with the knee bent slightly. The foot is turned outwards to laterally rotate the tibia under the femur. (This takes the tension off the lateral collateral ligament). 80% of body weight should be supported by the uninjured side.

Procedure:

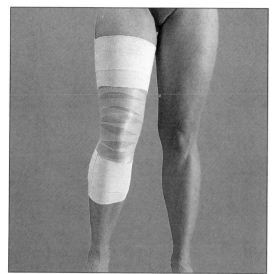

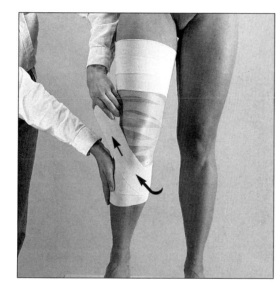

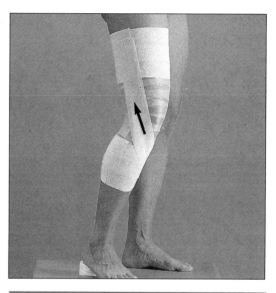

1. *Clean, shave and dry the skin to be taped checking for cuts, abrasions and sensitive areas.*
2. *Apply skin toughener, skin lubricant pads, prowrap and anchors as illustrated in previous technique. **For more detail, see steps 2,3,4,5 of MCL Taping page 133.***

TIP: Apply lubricant and padding on both hamstring tendons to protect tender skin from irritations, blisters and tape cuts.

3. *Begin the lateral lateral 7.5 cm (3 inch) elastic adhesive tape **X** with a strip starting anteriorly on the distal anchor, pulling up strongly around the tibia, and lateral to the patella finishing on the proximal anchor posteriorly.*

TIP: For stability, have the athlete place his hand on the taper's shoulder or use a nearby wall or other stable structure for support during the taping procedure – particulary during application of the lateral support arrows

NOTE: Be sure to maintain the knee in as much valgus as possible in order to keep the lateral aspect shortened

Knee Sprain (LCL)

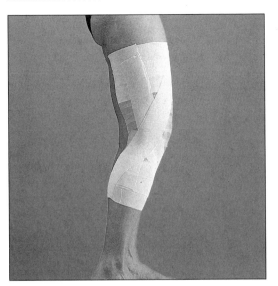

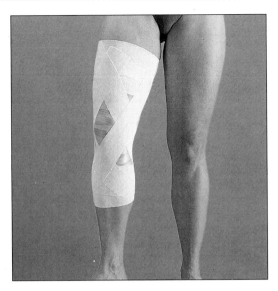

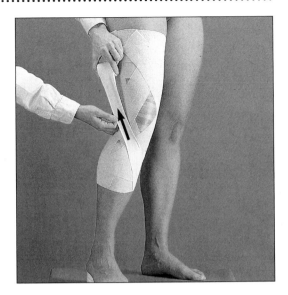

4. Complete the lateral **X** with a strip from the posteriolateral distal anchor, pulling up strongly to the anteriolateral proximal anchor, with the **X** over the lateral joint line.

5. Repeat anchor **X** on the medial aspect without causing internal rotation of the tibia or varus (outward) stress on the knee.

NOTE: Avoid compressing the patella when taping.

6. Use a vertical strip of white 5 cm (2 in.) tape with the edges folded in for extra strength, to reinforce the lateral ligament. Start anteriorly on the inferior anchor, and pull up strongly on the lateral side, keeping the knee in maximum varus and adhere the tape securely to the proximal anchor posteriorly.

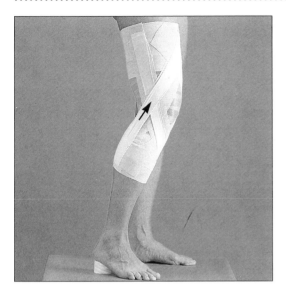

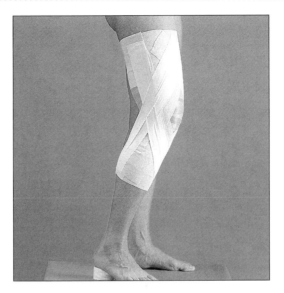

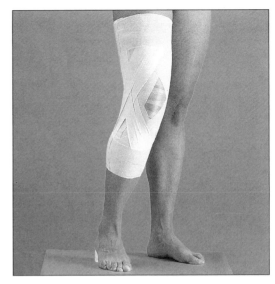

7. *Complete this laterally reinforcing **X** with a second vertical strip starting posteriorly on the distal anchor, and crossing the previous strip at the joint line. Maintain maximal varus while adhering the end to the proximal anchor anteriorly.*

NOTE: It is important to place these crosses over the lateral joint line well behind the patella.

8. *Apply the second white tape **X** slightly posterior to the first, with the **X** at the joint line.*

9. *Remember the tape job.*
10. *Before applying elastic wrap, test for degree of restriction:*
    a. extension must be restricted by 10°
    b. there must be no lateral laxity and
    c. there must be no pain on lateral stress testing (bending outwards) or extension.
11. ***Continue with steps 16, 18 &19 in the previous (MCL) taping page 140***

NOTES:
• For acute sprains: leave elastic wrap on for at least the first 48 hours.
• For back to sport taping, leave elastic wrap on for at least 15 minutes and remove for full activity.

Knee Sprain (LCL)

ANATOMICAL AREA: KNEE AND THIGH

INJURY: KNEE SPRAIN: LATERAL COLLATERAL LIGAMENT (LCL)

T ERMINOLOGY:
- lateral collateral ligament sprain
- external collateral ligament sprain
- fibular collateral ligament sprain
- torsion injury
- **see sprains chart page 36 for description 1st to 3rd degree of severity**

E TIOLOGY:
- excessive outward pressure forcing the knee laterally into varus (outwardly bent or "bow-legged" position)
- sudden impact forcing body medially on fixed lower leg
- direct blow to side of knee
- isolated tears are uncommon

S YMPTOMS:
- pain, tenderness on lateral side (outside) of the knee
- swelling, possible bruising
- active movement testing: lateral pain on end-range extension
- passive movement testing: lateral pain on end-range extension
- resistance testing (neutral position): no pain on moderate resistance
- stress testing at 0° and 30° knee flexion
  - **a.** 1st and 2nd degree sprains: pain with or without instability
  - **b.** 3rd degree of severity: complete ligament rupture ("opens up"); can be less pain than with 2nd degree sprain. See notes re: degree of injury testing (page 142)
  - **c.** instability at 0° extension is indicative of a severe injury with posterior capsule involvement

T REATMENT:
Early:
- R.I.C.E.S.
- therapeutic modalities

NOTE: Surgery may be indicated for 3rd degree of severity.

- taping for **LCL Sprain taping, see page 142** (plus elastic wrap – first 48 hours)

Later:
- continued physiotherapy including:
  - therapeutic modalities
  - transverse friction massage
  - mobilizations if stiff post-immobilization
- flexibility exercises for quadriceps, hamstrings and gastrocnemeii
- strengthening of quadriceps, hamstrings and gastrocnemeus
- strengthening of quadriceps (isometric at first)
- gradual reintegration program with pain free taped support: **for LCL sprain taping see page 142**
- total rehabilitation program for range of motion, flexibility, strength, and proprioception
- bracing may be recommended for return to activity or for continued athletics if chronically unstable

S EQUELAE:
- lateral (varus) laxity
- rotational instability
- predisposition to lateral meniscal tears
- weakness of quadriceps
- inability to "cut" when running
- possible peroneal nerve damage
- degenerative arthritic changes

R.I.C.E.S. : Rest, Ice, Compress, Elevate, Support

TAPING FOR ANTERIOR CRUCIATE LIGAMENT (ACL) SPRAINS OF THE KNEE

Purpose:
- reinforces knee stability bilaterally and posteriorly
- prevents the last 20° of extension
- reduces anterior translation of the tibia under the femur
- allows almost full flexion and functional extension

Indications for use:
- anterior cruciate ligament sprains (acute, subacute and chronic)
- posterior capsular trauma
- hamstring strains

MATERIALS:

razor
skin toughener spray
prowrap
lubricant
padding for hamstring tendons
7.5 cm (3 in.) elastic adhesive tape
10 cm (4 in.) elastic adhesive tape
5 cm (2 in.) or 3.8 cm (1.5 in.) non-elastic white tape
15.2 cm (6 in.) elastic wrap

NOTES:
- If an acute ACL sprain is suspected, the athlete MUST NOT return to play even if the disability seems mild. (In 3rd degree ruptures, a "pop" is often felt)
- Be certain that the athlete is examined by a competent sports-medicine specialist to confirm the diagnosis based on:
  a. a positive anterior drawer sign (forward sliding of the tibia under the femur at 90° of knee flexion)
  b. a positive Lachman's test (forward gliding of the tibia at 20° of knee flexion)
  c. a positive pivot shift (subluxation then sudden reduction of the lateral tibial plateau when flexing the knee from full extension with internal rotation of the tibia and a valgus stress at the knee)
- Apply adequate lubricant and padding over both hamstring tendons to protect the tender skin in this area from irritation, blisters and tape cuts.

For additional details regarding an injury example see TESTS chart page 151.

Positioning:

Standing on a stool or chair with a roll of tape under the heel of the injured leg and the knee in 40° of flexion (weight is borne on both legs).

Procedure:

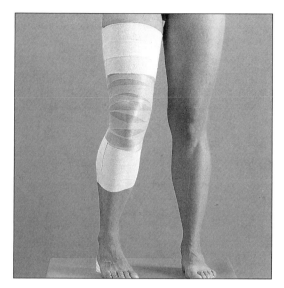

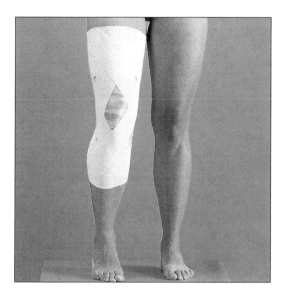

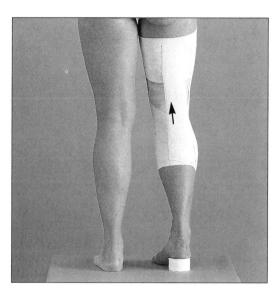

1. *Clean, shave and dry the skin to be taped, checking for cuts, abrasions, and sensitive areas.*
2. *Apply padding and lubricant to the popliteal fossa and hamstring tendons.*
3. *Apply skin toughener, prowrap and anchors as illustrated in the previous technique: **see steps 3, 4, 5 of MCL taping for more details: page 134**.*

4. *Apply a 7.5 cm (3 in.) elastic adhesive **X** over the medial joint line using moderate tension.*
5. *Repeat step 4 on the lateral side.*

6. *To form a check-rein, apply the first restraining strips vertically from the lower to the upper anchors with 7.5 cm (3 in.) elastic adhesive tape. Keep the knee flexed at least 40° and stretch this strip maximally between the anchors.*

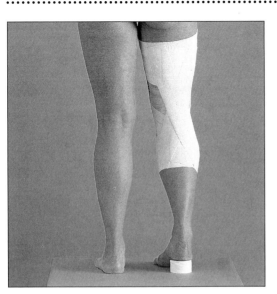

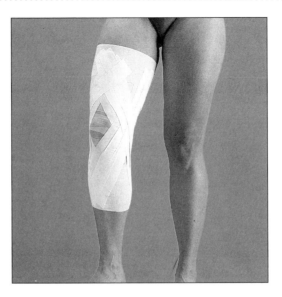

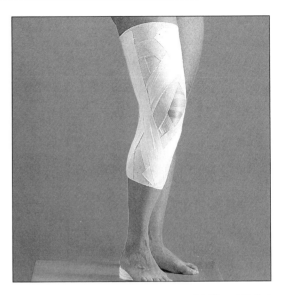

7. *Complete the posterior restraining strip with an* ***X*** *directly over the back of the knee.*

8. *Reanchor these strips with 10 cm (4 in.) elastoplast from mid-thigh to mid-calf.*

> **NOTE:** Enough tension must be used so that the completed taping will completely block at least the last 20° of knee extension when maximally stressed.

9. *Reinforce the medial elastic adhesive* ***X*** *with two 5 cm (2 in.) white tape* ***X*** *s, overlapping the second one slightly anteriorly to the first.*

10. *Reinforce the lateral elastic adhesive* ***X*** *in the same way.*

11. *Re-anchor*

12. *Before applying the elastic wrap, test the degree of restriction:*

a. *extension must be limited by at least 20°*

b. *there must be no pain on passive extension*

13. *Close and wrap the tape job as shown in* ***MCL Taping, Steps 16, 18, and 19.***

> **NOTE:**
> • For acute sprains, leave elastic wrap on for at least the first **48** hours.
> • For back to sport taping, leave elastic wrap on for at least **15** minutes and remove for full activity.

ANATOMICAL AREA: KNEE AND THIGH

INJURY: KNEE SPRAIN: ANTERIOR CRUCIATE LIGAMENT: ACL

T ERMINOLOGY:
- anterior cruciate ligament sprain: severity of 1st to 3rd degree (**see SPRAINS Chart, page 36**).
- hyperextension injury
- torsion injury

E TIOLOGY:
- forced anterior glide of the tibia under the femur
- forced hyperextension
- forward fall with foot fixed in position
- direct frontal blow

S YMPTOMS:
- often history of a "pop" sensation
- swelling
- active movement testing:
  a. decreased range of motion and pain on end-range extension, varying with severity
  b. decreased range and pain an extreme flexion in indicative of marked intra-articular swelling
- passive movement testing:
  a. pain on end-range extension with 1st and 2nd degree sprains;
  b. isolated 3rd degree may be pain-free
- resistance testing (neutral position): no pain on moderate resistance
- stress testing: positive "Lachman's" and lateral pivot shift tests: **see notes for ACL introduction page 148**.

T REATMENT:
Early:
- R.I.C.E.S.
- Taping for **ACL sprain taping, see page 148** (plus elastic wrap – first 48 hrs.)
- therapeutic modalities

> NOTE: Surgery often recommended for 3rd degree of severity.

Later:
- continued physiotherapy including:
  - therapeutic modalities
  - avoidance of terminal knee extension initially
  - specific strengthening of hamstring muscles
  - gradual pain-free return to sports activity with taped support as above. (**For ACL Sprain taping, see page 148**)
- total rehabilitation program for range of motion, flexibility, strength and proprioception
- may require bracing

S EQUELAE:
- chronic pain
- instability
- "giving way"; "trick" knee
- predisposition to meniscal injuries
- weakness of quadriceps
- degenerative arthritic changes

R.I.C.E.S. : Rest, Ice, Compress, Elevate, Support

Knee Sprain (ACL)

TAPING FOR PATELLO-FEMORAL PAIN

Purpose:
- compresses the patella tendon thereby changing lines of stress and thus altering the biomechanics of the patello-femoral joint
- reduces upward mobility of patella
- allows full movement at the knee joint.

Indications for use:
- patellar tendinitis
- patello-femoral pain syndrome
- Osgood-Schlatter's disease
- medial knee pain associated with flat feet
- "jumper's knee"

MATERIALS:

razor
quick drying adhesive spray
2.5 cm (1 in.) semi-elastic tape (preferable) or non-elastic white tape
(semi-elastic tape: has a minimal amount of elasticity and is not a conventional elastic adhesive tape)

NOTES:
- Evaluate pain on a scale of 0 to 10 with 0 being nil and 10 being the worst pain, prior to taping, by having the athlete perform a half-squat. Re-evaluate this movement throughout the taping procedure, monitoring any change in pain. Use only the taping strips which alleviate the pain.
- Avoid compressing the patella against the femur, as this may aggravate pain.
- There should be no pain during activity. Should the athlete NOT be able to function pain-free, McConnell* techniques may be indicated.
- The semi-elastic adhesive tape used in this procedure is minimally elastic and maximally adherent. Should it not be available, use white adhesive tape instead (do not use elastic adhesive tape).

* See reference, page 223.

For additional details regarding an injury see TESTS chart page 156

Positioning:

Relaxed, supported long sitting position or supine, with the knee aligned in a neutral position and supported on a roll or cushion.

Procedure:

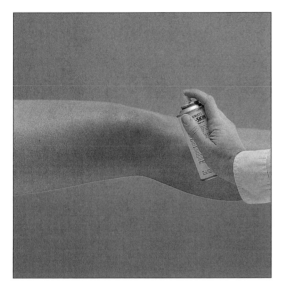

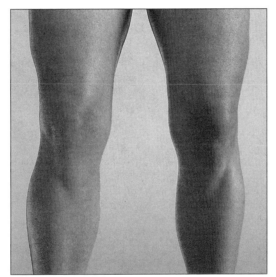

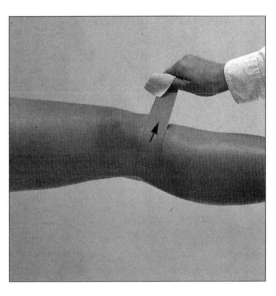

1. Clean, shave and dry the area to be taped, checking for cuts, abrasions and sensitive areas.

2. Spray liberally with quick dry adhesive spray and let dry completely.

3. Perform the test position: a half-squat with weight more on the painful leg.

NOTE: Assess the intensity of pain, and the knee angle at pain onset.

4. Starting posteriorly on the lateral side, apply a horizontal strip of 2.5 cm (1 in.) semi-elastic adhesive tape. Using moderately firm pressure this strip should compress the patellar tendon just above the tibial tubercle .

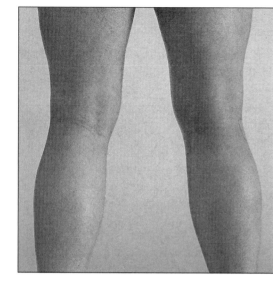

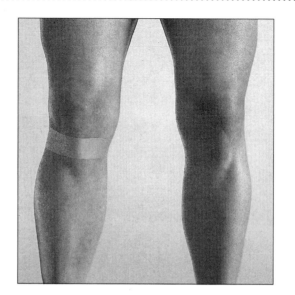

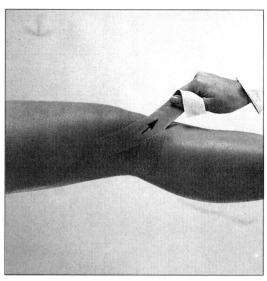

5. *Re-evaluate the level of pain.*

6. *Apply a diagonal strip of tape from the upper lateral aspect of the knee beside the patella, pulling distally across the patellar tendon ending medially.*

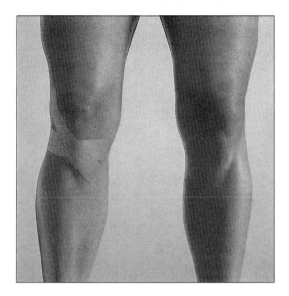

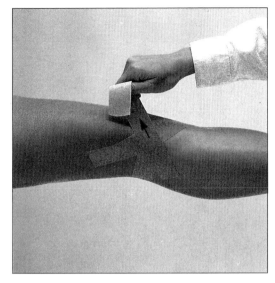

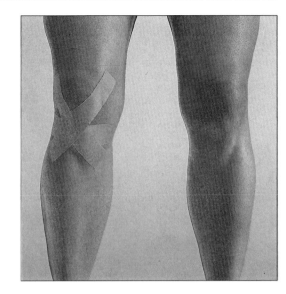

7. Re-evaluate the level of pain.

8. Apply a diagonal strip of tape from the lower lateral aspect of the knee beside the patella, pulling proximally across the patellar tendon ending medially.

9. Re-evaluate the level of pain.

a. 40° of full weightbearing flexion should be possible.

b. If pain is not eliminated with this taping, try McConnell taping combined with her biomechanically corrective approach. (See reference page 223.)

NOTE: Active physiotherapy should precede returning to activity.

ANATOMICAL AREA: KNEE AND THIGH

CONDITION: PATELLO-FEMORAL SYNDROME

T ERMINOLOGY:
- patellar alignment syndrome
- retro-patellar inflammation
- pre-chondromalacia

E TIOLOGY:
- quadriceps weakness
- poor tracking of patella
- subluxing or dislocating patella
- poor biomechanics of adjacent joints
- post-traumatic blow to knee
- secondary to patellar tendinitis
- jumping as in plyometric training
- common in basketball and volleyball

S YMPTOMS:
- peripatellar pain may be experienced in various locations:
  a. diffuse around the patella (knee cap)
  b. at the inferior tip of the patella
  c. anterior or posterior to the patellar tendon
  d. at the tibial tubercle (insertion of the tendon)
- pain is often felt following sitting or resting
- active movement testing: may have pain on extension; pain when climbing or particularly when descending stairs
- passive movement testing: muscle tightness or imbalance involving quadriceps, hamstrings and tensor fascia lata (TFL)
- resistance testing (neutral position): weakness of quadriceps (specifically vastus medialis obligus [VMO]) with or without pain
- stress testing: patello-femoral grinding test causes pain

T REATMENT:
Early:
(if acutely inflamed)
- ice
- therapeutic modalities
- lateral retinacular stretching
- taping: **for Patellar Tendon taping** *see* **page 152**.

NOTE: If pain is not eliminated with this taping, try McConnell taping combined with her treatment protocol. See reference no. 16 page 223.

Later:
- continued physiotherapy including:
  - therapeutic modalities to control pain
  - quadriceps re-education: particularly vastus medialis obliqus (VMO) utilizing muscle stimulation or biofeedback
  - flexibility exercises, hamstring and tensor fascia lata (TFL)
- gradually progressive negative weight-training with corrected biomechanics (proper patellar tracking) and taping. (**for Patellar Tendon taping,** *see* **page 152**)
- orthiotics may help if faulty alignment is caused by poor foot biomechanics.

S EQUELAE:
- chronic pain of quadriceps
- weakness of quadriceps and tensor fascia lata (TFL)
- inflexibility
- inability to participate in sports
- chondromalacia

TAPING FOR QUADRICEPS (THIGH) CONTUSION OR STRAIN

Purpose:
- applies localized specific compression to the bruised or torn tissue
- prevents subsequent swelling, bleeding or muscle fibre tearing in the area
- allows full function and flexibility

Indications for use:
- quadriceps contusion ("charley-horse")
- quadriceps strain
- for hamstring strains tape is applied to posterior thigh

MATERIALS:

razor
skin toughener spray
10 cm (4 in.) elastic adhesive tape
7.5 cm (3 in.) elastic adhesive tape
3.8 cm (1.5 in.) non-elastic white tape
15.2 cm (6 in.) elastic wrap

NOTES:
- The exact site of the contusion or strain must be localized.
- Prowrap is not recommended, as it significantly lessens the effectiveness of the tape technique.
- The pressure of tape strips must be localized to the injured area and not too tight cicumferentially. If constricted, hamstring and calf muscles may cramp; as well, the athlete may feel that the leg is weak, stiff or heavy.
- Icing and gentle stretching of the injured muscle should start immediately.
- Any massage is strictly contraindicated in the early stages due to the high risk of further internal bleeding and the potential development of myocytis ossificans.

For additional details regarding an injury example see TESTS chart page 164.

Positioning:

Lying on a bench with the knee flexed over the edge, and the heel resting on the ground or the floor.

Procedure:

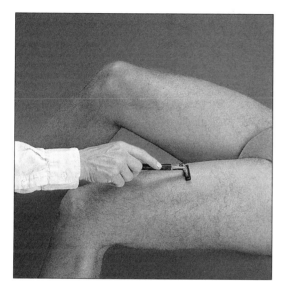

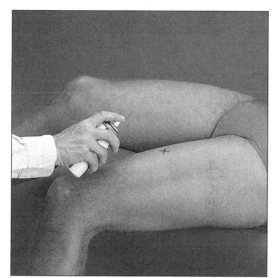

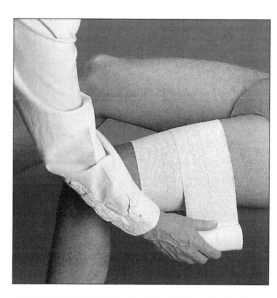

1. Clean, shave and dry the area to be taped, checking for cuts, abrasions and sensitive areas.

2. Localize and mark the exact site of the contusion or muscle strain.
3. Spray quick dry adhesive circumferentially to the thigh and let dry completely.

4. Begin 7.6 cm (3 in.) below the lower aspect of the injury, wrap 10 cm (4 in.) elastic adhesive tape around the limb using light tension. Repeat this strip overlapping the previous one by 1.5 cm (5/8 in.) until the entire injured area is covered and surpassed by 7.5 cm (3 in.)

NOTE: This layer of tape forms a foundation for the compression strips to avoid excessive tension on the skin.

Quadraceps Contusion

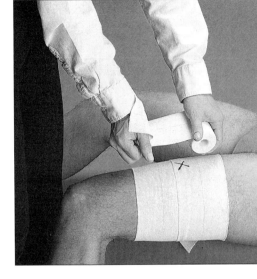

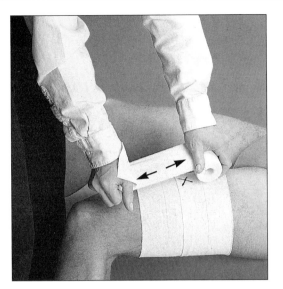

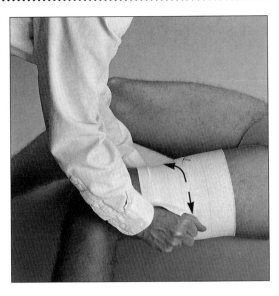

NOTE: For large thighs or large contusions, 10 cm (4 in.) tape can be used for these strips if the taper has wide enough hands to maintain pressure across the entire tape width.

5. Prepare to apply the first pressure strip directly below the centre of the site of injury.

a. Fold back 12 cm (5 in.) at the end of a roll of 7.5 cm (3 in.) elastic adhesive tape in one hand and hold the remainder of the roll in the other.

5b. Stretch the tape fully, holding the tape horizontally, across the limb and keep it stretched laterally.

5c. Apply strong pressure to the limb equally with both hands while maintaining lateral stretch until the tape reaches 3/4 of the way around the limb. Wrap the tape ends towards the back and let the roll hang down on the medial side.

NOTE: This usually causes some discomfort.

TIP: The taper can better stabilize and control counterpressure by gripping and squeezing the athlete's knee with their own knees to gain better support during the application of the pressure strips. (Technique not illustrated.)

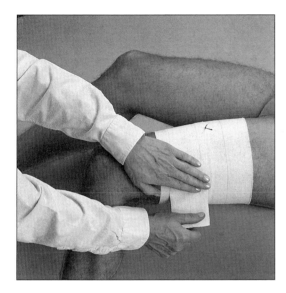

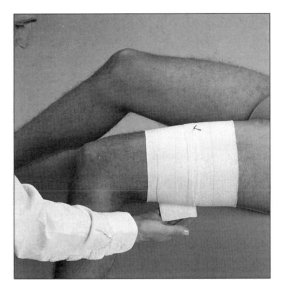

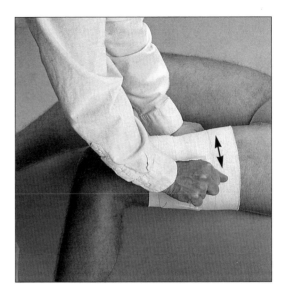

5d. *Be careful to keep the strip from detaching and release the tension completely before adhering the lateral tape end posteriorly.*

5e. *Complete encircling the limb by overlapping tape ends well at the back without tension..*

TIP: Ensure the medial side does not detatch while cutting the tape from the roll.

6. *Repeat the pressure strip overlapping by half the tape's width above the last strip proximally, focussing the pressure directly over the lower half of the injury.*

7. *Repeat again directly over the injury always with maximal pressure anteriorly.*

NOTE: This will be quite painful when pressure is applied directly to the injury site.

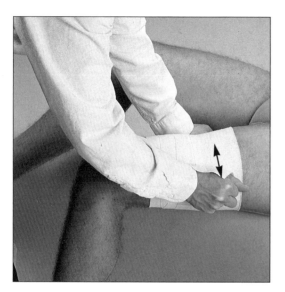

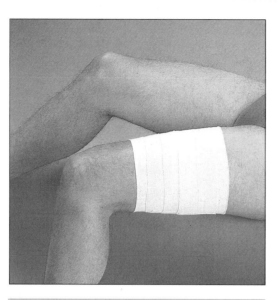

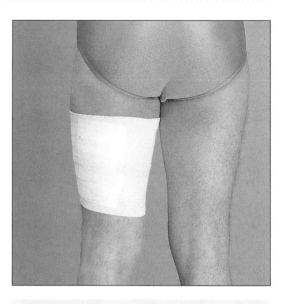

8. *Continue repeating the pressure strips overlapping by 1/2 more proximally until the entire tape base is covered.*

TIP: Ensure that the tape job extends at least one full tape-width higher and lower than the area of injury.

9. *Finish the ends of this taping with short strips of white tape to avoid detachment of the elastic tape while in action.*

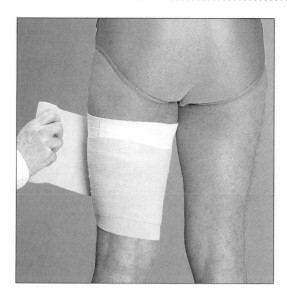

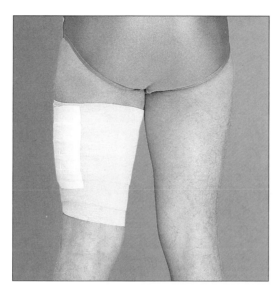

10. Wrap the entire tape job with an elastic wrap, prior to activity, to give the adhesive in the tape the time and heat necessary in order to set (remove prior to playing).

11. Affix the elastic wrap with white tape.
12. Reassess the degree of pain
  a. isometrically
  b. dynamically

NOTE: Prevention of further bleeding and maintenance of full muscle flexibility are critical for rapid recovery.

TIP: Because maintaining full flexibility is critical, an elastic wrap should be used to attach an ice pack to the thigh while keeping the knee fully flexed. (The bandage encircles the ice pack, thigh and lower leg simultaneously.)

ANATOMICAL AREA: KNEE AND THIGH

CONDITION: QUADRICEPS CONTUSION

T ERMINOLOGY:
- contusion of one of the quadriceps muscles 1st to 3rd degree severity (**See CONTUSION Chart see page 38.**)
- "charley-horse"

E TIOLOGY:
- direct blow on thigh (example: a puck forcefully hitting the thigh in ice hockey; or a direct hit to the thigh in rugby or football)

S YMPTOMS:
- pain, tenderness over site of injury
- swelling and haematoma if not treated immediately
- active movement testing: pain on active contraction of quadriceps
- passive movement testing:
  a. pain on knee flexion
  b. worse with hip extension
- resistance testing (neutral position): pain and/or weakness of quadriceps
- palpable localized deformity possible

T REATMENT:
Early:
- ICE!
- taping: **for Compression taping see page 158**.
- early flexibility exercises enhanced by active contraction of hamstrings only; no over-pressure
- therapeutic modalities
- gentle activity with taped compression

Later:
- continued physiotherapy including:
  - therapeutic modalities
  - strengthening exercises: pain-free
  - flexibility exercises
- gradual return to full pain-free activity with taped support. For **Compression taping: see page 158**.
- dynamic proprioceptive program

NOTE: A dense foam pad reinforced with a hard outer shell will protect area from further injury.

S EQUELAE:
- haematoma
- myositis ossificans if massaged early
- complete rupture of muscle if used too early
- weakness
- scarring and inflexibility
- predisposition to recurrent strains

ANATOMICAL AREA: KNEE AND THIGH

TAPING FOR ADDUCTOR (GROIN) STRAIN TAPING:

Purpose:
- applies localized support and compression over the injured muscles
- allows full flexion and extension
- applies local pressure while permitting full flexibility
- can be adapted to also restrict abduction

Indications for use:
- acute adductor (groin) strain
- chronic adductor (groin) strain
- adductor tendinitis

MATERIALS:

razor
skin toughener spray
10 cm (4 in.) elastic adhesive tape
7.5 cm (3 in.) elastic adhesive tape
3.8 cm (1.5 in.) non-elastic white tape
15.2 cm (6 in.) elastic wrap

NOTES:
- The exact site of the injury must be localized.
- Be certain that groin injuries of the muscle attachments at the pubic bone are evaluated by a physician.
- X-rays should be taken to rule out avulsion or stress fractures.
- The skin near the groin is extremely tender and prone to irritation: careful preparation of the area is essential.
- Once taped, the usual pre-event stretches must not be omitted. Proper flexibility will reduce the risk of reinjury or an increase in the severity of the current injury.

For additional details regarding an injury example see TESTS chart page 170

Positioning:

Standing on a stool with knee slightly bent, the heel resting on a roll of tape, and foot turned inwards. (This decreases the stretch of the groin muscles.)

Recheck this position frequently during the course of the taping.

Procedure:

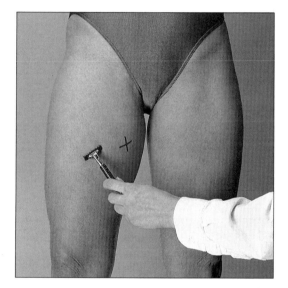

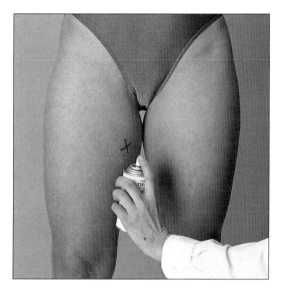

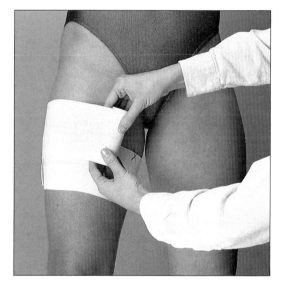

1. Clean, shave and dry the skin to be taped, checking for cuts, abrasions and sensitive areas.

2. Localize and mark the exact site of the injury.
3. Spray skin toughener over the thigh circumferentially, to enhance adherence and to protect the skin from irritation.

4. Apply one layer of 10 cm (4 in.) elastic adhesive tape with light tension around the limb.
5. Continue additional foundation strips overlapping by 2 - 3 cm (.5 in. –1 in.) until the tape covers an area at least 7.6 cm (3 in.) above and below the injury site.

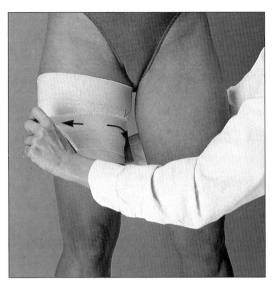

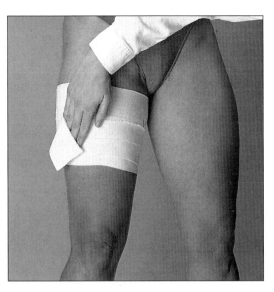

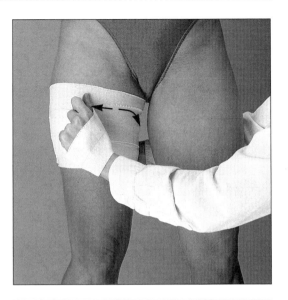

6. *Apply the first pressure strip slightly below the site of injury.*

a. *First stretch the tape fully and then apply it with strong pressure equally with both hands. Release the pressure only when the tape strip reaches 3/4 of the way around the leg.*

6b. *Apply the remainder of the strip ends encircling the limb with little or no tension, being careful not to allow these to peel back and consequently lose the localized pressure.*

7. *Apply subsequent strips of tape proximally, overlapping by one half the width of the tape above this first strip, as in the previous technique (see pages 160–162)*

NOTE: The finished tape job should have no creases or folds.

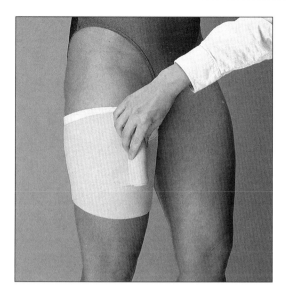

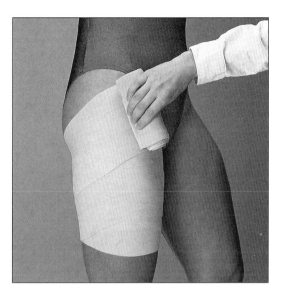

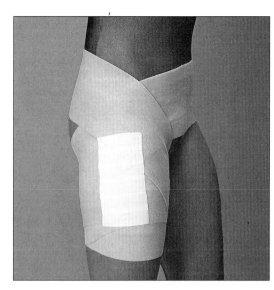

8. Cover the ends of this taping with short strips of white tape.

9. Wrap the entire tape job with an elastic bandage to allow the adhesive in the tape time and heat necessary in order to set, in the following fashion (the hip spica technique).

a. Wrap the tensor in a modified figure-8 medially around the upper thigh,

9b. then around the hip and waist.

TIP: Maintain correct positioning in slight internal rotation.

10. Affix the end of the wrap with white non-elastic tape.

11. Test the degree of pain reduction

a. isometrically

b. dynamically

NOTE: This "spica" elastic wrap can be reinforced with a second wrap pulled tightly enough to assist adduction and restrict abduction.

ANATOMICAL AREA: KNEE AND THIGH

INJURY: ADDUCTOR STRAIN

T ERMINOLOGY:
- strain of one of the adductor muscle or tendons, severity: 1st to 3rd degree. **(See STRAIN Chart page 37).**
- "pulled" groin muscle

E TIOLOGY:
- explosive contraction of adductor muscles
- excessive stretch of adductor muscles
- more susceptible when muscles are not warmed up
- overuse due to unaccustomed repetitive action
- common in goal-tending, soccer, hockey, football and some track and field sports.

S YMPTOMS:
- slight to severe pain varying with degree and location of injury
- pain may be diffuse or localized and may reach as high as pubic bone
- haematoma not always present
- active movement testing:
  a. some pain on hip adduction
  b. pain also possible on active abduction due to muscle stretch.
- passive movement testing: pain on hip adduction
- resistance testing (neutral position: pain and/or weakness on hip adduction

> NOTE: Although an avulsion of the inferior pubic ramus (pubic bone chip) at the muscle insertion is rare, it should be ruled out by X-ray if the pain is localized and persistent.

T REATMENT:
Early:
- R.I.C.E.S.
- taping: for **Adductor Strain taping see page 166.**
- therapeutic modalities

Later:
- continued physiotherapy including:
  - transverse friction massage
  - progressive, graduated exercises to regain strength (isometric and non-weightbearing at first)
- gradual reintegration to activities program with pain-free taped support; **(For Adductor Strain taping see page 166.)**

S EQUELAE:
- persistent pain
- weakness
- scarring and inflexibility
- chronic reinjury
- imbalance may lead to pelvic and lumbar spine compensatory problems
- bone spurs may develop
- ossification of haematoma possible

R.I.C.E.S. : Rest, Ice, Compress, Elevate, Support

Chapter Eight ....

SHOULDER AND ELBOW

The **gleno-humeral** (shoulder) joint is the most mobile of all the joints in the human body. It is this mobility that predisposes the shoulder to instability - both acute and chronic - and heightens the joint's dependency on muscular and capsular support. By contrast, the adjacent **acromio-clavicular** (A/C) joint, is less mobile and depends solely on ligaments for support. In this section, two techniques useful in preventing post-injury damage to this vulnerable joint system are demonstrated.

At the elbow, the **humero-ulnar** joint (the true elbow joint), is a hinge joint like the knee. It sustains some similar injuries, requiring the application of taping principles presented in the knee/thigh section.

The main purpose and value in taping an elbow is the prevention of full extension of the joint, with or without lateral reinforcement. Because the associated **radio-ulnar** (forearm) joints allow a great degree of pronation and supination (rotation) the overall effectiveness of taping for lateral ligaments is compromised.

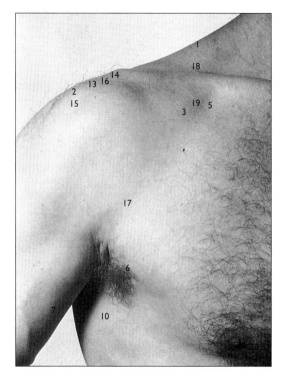

MUSCLES
1. TRAPEZIUS
2. DELTOID
3. ANTERIOR MARGIN OF DELTOID
4. PECTORALIS MAJOR
5. UPPER MARGIN PECTORALIS MAJOR
6. LOWER MARGIN PECTORALIS MAJOR
7. BICEPS SHORT HEAD
8. CORACO BRACHIALIS
9. TERES MAJOR
10. SERRATUS ANTERIOR
11. TRICEPS
TENDONS
12. LATISSIMUS DORSI
BONES
13. ACROMION OF SCAPULA
14. ACROMAL END OF CLAVICLES
15. GREATER TUBEROSITY OF HUMERUS
JOINTS
16. ACROMIOCLAVICULAR
HOLLOWS
17. DELTO PECTORAL GROOVE
18. SUPRA CLAVICULAR FOSSA
19. INFRA CLAVICULAR FOSSA
MISCELLANEOUS
20. AREOLA
21. NIPPLE

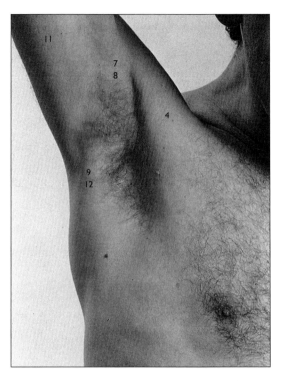

Right shoulder from the front
The arm is slightly abducted
- The nipple in the male (21) normally lies at the level of the fourth intercostal space.
- The deltopectoral groove containing the cephalic vein is formed by the adjacent borders of deltoid (2) and pectoralis major (5).
- The lower border of pectoralis major (6) forms the anterior fold.

The right axilla or armpit is the hollow below the shoulder. Its anterior wall is made up mainly of fibres of pectoralis major (4) with pectoralis minor behind. The posterior wall consists of teres major (9) with the tendon of latissimus dorsi (12) immediately in front. Close to pectoralis major a bundle of muscle made up of the short head of biceps (7) and coracobrachialis (8) runs down the arm with the cords of the brachial plexus surrounding the axillary artery immediately behind. The axilla is also a very important site for lymph glands draining lymphatics from the arm and most importantly the breast.

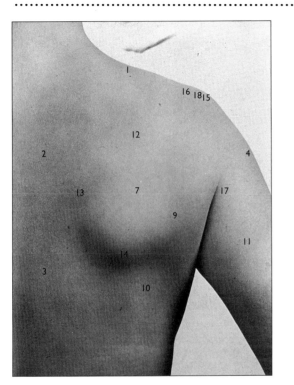

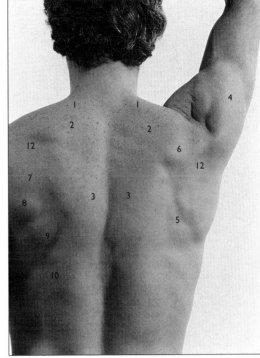

MUSCLES
1   TRAPEZIUS - UPPER FIBRES
2   TRAPEZIUS - MIDDLE FIBRES
3   TRAPEZIUS - LOWER FIBRES
4   DELTOID
5   RHOMBOIDEUS MAJOR
6   SUPRA SPINATUS
7   INFRA SPINATUS
8   TERES MINOR
9   TERES MAJOR
10 LATISSIMUS DORSI
11 TRICEPS
BONES
12 SPINE OF SCAPULA
13 VERTEBRAL BORDER OF SCAPULA
14 INFERIOR ANGLUS OF SCAPULA
15 ACROMION OF SCAPULA
16 ACROMIAL END OF CLAVICLE
NERVES
17 AXILLARY NERVES POSTERIOR TO HUMERUS
JOINTS
18 ACROMIO-CAVICULAR

Right shoulder, from behind.

The arm is slightly abducted and the inferior angle of the scapula (14) has been made to project backwards by attempting to flex the shoulder joint against resistance.

- The inferior angle of the scapula (14) usually lies at the level of the seventh intercostal space. It is overlapped by the upper margin of latissimus dorsi (10).
- The axillary nerve (17) runs transversely under cover of deltoid (4) behind the shaft of the humerus at a level 5 to 6 cm below the acromion (15).
- Latissimus dorsi (10) and teres major (9) form the lower boundary of the posterior wall of the axilla.

Right shoulder, arm elevated:

While maintaining good postural control of the trunk the right arm has been abducted through some 180°. The left scapula remains in a normal resting position but with firm muscle control, the glenoid pointing laterally. The right scapula has been rotated through some 70–75° under the activity of trapezius with the remaining arm movement occurring at the shoulder joint. Activity is obvious in deltoid (4) the major abductor at the shoulder joint, and no doubt in supraspinatus (6), though this muscle is masked by trapezius (2).

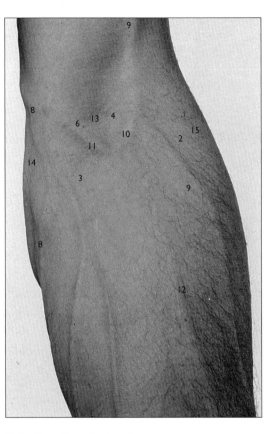

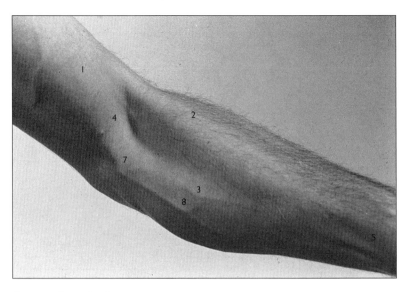

Forearm from the front

Left elbow from the front

There is an M-shaped pattern of superficial veins cephalic (9) and basilic (8) veins are joined by a median cubital vein into which drain two small median forearm veins

The order of the structures in the cubital fossa from lateral to medial is biceps tendon (4) brachial artery (13) and median nerve (6).

MUSCLES	10 MEDIAN CEPHALIC VEIN
1 BICEPS	11 MEDIAN BASILIC VEIN
2 BRACHIO RADIALIS	12 MEDIAN FOREARM VEIN
3 PRONATOR TERES	**ARTERIES**
4 BICEPS	13 BRACHIAL
5 FLEXOR CARPI RADIALIS	**BONES**
NERVES	14 MEDIAL EPICONDYLE OF HUMERUS
6 MEDIAN	15 LATERAL EPICONDYLE OF HUMERUS
FASCIA	
7 BICIPITAL APONEUROSIS	
VEINS	
8 BASILIC	
9 CEPHALIC VEIN	

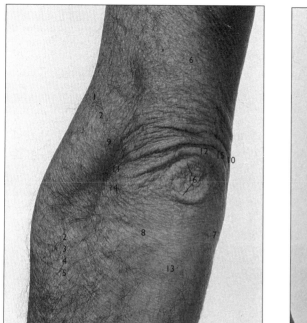

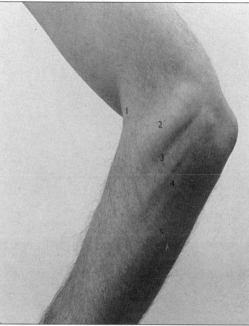

The back of the forearm

The superficial extensor muscles take a common origin from the lateral epicondyle of the humerus (9) and the supracondylar ridge. Brachioradialis (1), the muscle coming from higher up the ridge, has been described with the anterior muscles in view of its flexor role. *Extensor carpi radialis longus* (2) also comes from the supracondylar ridge below brachioradialis and, below that, *extensor carpi radialis brevis* (3) arises from the epicondyle. These three muscles can usually be identified, quite easily, running down the radial side of the back of the forearm.

Left elbow, from behind.

With the elbow fully extended, the extensor muscles form a bulge on the lateral side. In the adjacent hollow can be felt the head of the radius (14) and the capitulum of the humerus (11) which indicate the line of the humeroradial part of the elbow joint. The lateral and medial epicondyles of the humerus (9 and 10) are palpable on each side. Wrinkled skin lies at the back of the prominent olecranon of the ulna (12), and in this arm the margin of the olecranon bursa (16) is outlined. The most important structure in this region is the ulnar nerve (15) which is palpable as it lies in contact with the humerus behind the medial epicondyle (10). The posterior border of the ulna (13) is subcutaneous throughout its whole length

- With the elbow extended (straight) the medial and lateral epicondyles of the humerus (10 and 9) and the olecranon of the ulna (12) are on the same level, but with flexion of the elbow the olecranon moves to a lower level.
- The subcutaneous position of the ulnar nerve (15) behind the medial epicondyle of the humerus (10) makes it easily palpable: here it can be rolled against bone or injured with paraesthesia (tingling sensation) in the distribution of the nerve on the ulnar side of the hand.
- The region of the medial epicondyle of the humerus is referred to as the "funny bone"

MUSCLES
1 BRACHIO RADIALIS
2 EXTENSOR CARPI RADIALIS LONGUS
3 EXTENSOR CARPI RADIALIS BREVIS
4 EXTENSOR DIGITORUM
5 EXTENSOR CARPI ULNARIS
6 TRICEPS
7 FLEXOR CARPI ULANARIS
8 ANCONEUS
BONES
9 LATERAL EPICONDYLE OF HUMEROUS
10 MEDIAL EPICONDYLE OF HUMEROUS
11 CAPITULUM OF HUMEROUS
12 OLECRANON OF ULNA
13 POSTERIOR BORDER OF ULNA
14 HEAD OF RADIUS
NERVES
15 ULNAR
BURSA
16 MARGIN OF OLECRONON BURSA

TAPING FOR ACROMIO-CLAVICULAR (A/C): SHOULDER SEPARATION

Purpose:
- compresses and stabilizes the acromio-clavicular (A/C) joint.
- keeps the distal end of the clavicle down while allowing almost full gleno-humeral function.
- elastic support assists abduction.

Indications for use:
- acute A/C sprain
- sub-acute shoulder separation
- chronic shoulder separation
- chronic step deformity accompanied by pain at the A/C joint

TIP: Ensure that step deformity is corrected/reduced by proper positioning.

NOTES:
- Acutely injured athletes should not return to competition without proper investigation. (High risk of advancing severity of the injury.)
- Ensure correct diagnosis by following up with a sports-medicine specialist.
- Be certain that a radiological evaluation is done, particularly if any deformity is present.
- This taping can be used for a female athlete by applying the chest anchors below the breasts, and the anterior end of the vertical anchor angled more toward midline.
- Monitor limb sensation, strength of pulse and venous return prior to, during and after taping to ensure that there is no neurovascular compromise.
- Tender skin at the axilla (armpit) needs special attention and protection.

MATERIALS:

rectangular piece of felt or very dense foam approximately 5 x 3.6 cm (2 x 1.4 in.) and 1 cm (0.4 in.) thick to cover A/C joint
square of gauze, thin felt or folded prowrap approximately 3.6 x 3.6 cm (2 in. sq.) to cover nipple
razor
skin toughener spray
3.8 cm (1.5 in.) white tape
7.5 cm (3 in.)elastic adhesive tape
5 cm (2 in.) elastic adhesive tape

For additional details regarding an injury example see TESTS chart page 182.

Positioning:

Sitting comfortably with the elbow and forearm well supported across the lap with a solid cushion.

Procedure:

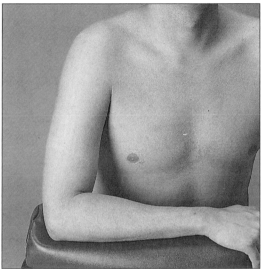

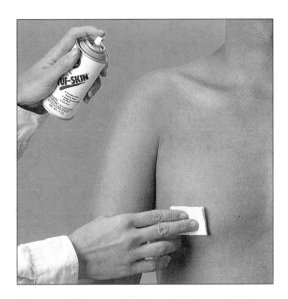

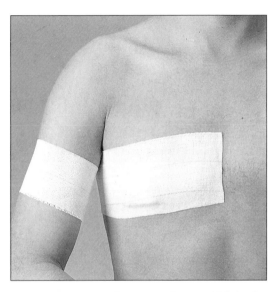

1. *Clean skin thoroughly and check for any abrasions, cuts, or sensitive areas.*
2. *Shave the upper arm and chest area in a 15 cm (6 in.) strip.*

NOTE: sensation, pulse, temperature and colour must be checked before starting to tape.

3. *Spray the area well with **tape adherent** to maximize adhesiveness thus stabilizing anchors.*

TIP: Turn athlete's face away and protect nipple when spraying.

4. *Wrap an anchor with light tension around mid-humerus with 7.5 cm (3 in.) elastic adhesive tape.*

TIP: Ensure that the last 7.5 cm (3 in.) the ends of the anchors are applied without tension and pressed firmly to avoid "peeling back" of the tape.

5. *Apply two anchors of 7.5 cm (3 in.) elastic adhesive tape horizontally to the chest with light pressure, from anterior to posterior at the level of the 5th rib (covering the nipple with gauze, prowrap or felt).*

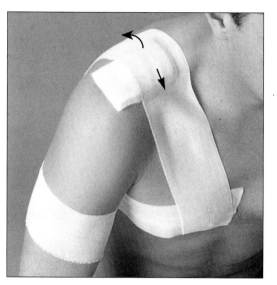

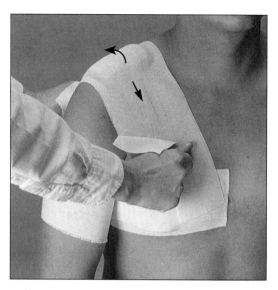

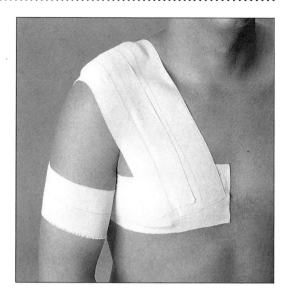

6. *Cut a piece of felt or dense foam padding large enough to cover the prominence of the A/C joint. (approx. 3.5 x 5 cm [1¹/2 x 2 in.] and at least 1 cm [0.4 in.] thick).*

7. *Using 7.5 cm (3 in.) elastic adhesive tape and moderate tension, apply rectangle directly on the upper end of the A/C joint (outer tip of the clavicle and adjacent acromion).*

TIP: Be sure the athlete is still sitting well-positioned with the forearm supported.

8. *Apply a compression strip of tape directly downwards over the distal end of the clavicle. Extend the elastic tape horizontally as much as possible and apply through the padding with strong pressure downwards while maintaining the horizontal tension. Release the tension only when the ends of the strip reach the chest anchor anteriorly and posteriorly (front and back).*

TIP: Ensure that the last 7.5 cm (3 in.) of tape is completely without tension when being affixed.

9. *Repeat this strip, moving laterally to cover one half of the first strip.*

NOTE: Recheck sensation, pulse, temperature, colour.

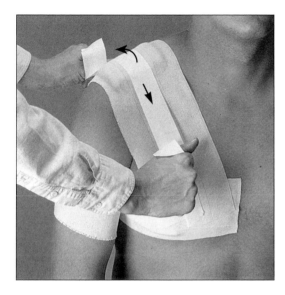

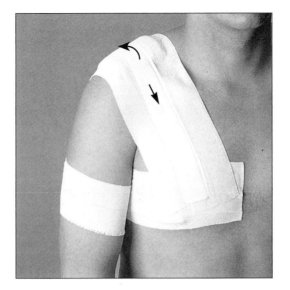

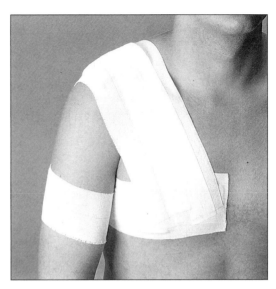

10. *Reinforce stability by applying a strip of 3.8 cm (1.5 inch) white tape:*

a. *Maintain strong horizontal tension while applying strong pressure downwards on the superior (upper) aspect of the A/C padding.*

TIP: Do not release tension until the anchors are reached.

10b. *Ensure that these strips cross the anchor completely.*

11. *Apply a second downwards strip of white tape more laterally.*

NOTE: These strips further stabilize distal end of clavicle and approximate normal anatomical position of the joint.

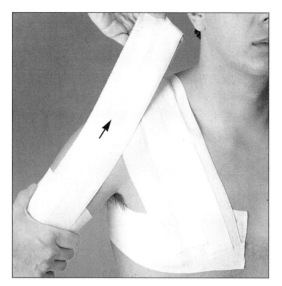

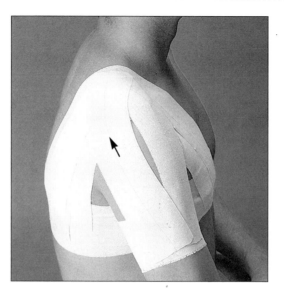

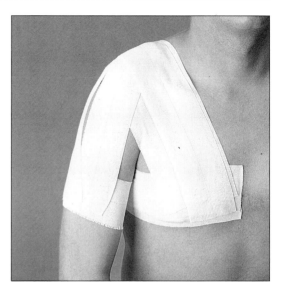

12. With the arm in a 45° angle of abduction, place a strip of 7.5 cm (3 in.) elastic adhesive tape starting laterally from the arm anchor going anteriorly across the top of the padding pulling up with firm tension to take the weight of the arm off the distal part of the joint.

13. Repeat this strip starting posterolaterally on the arm and pulling up on the posterior aspect of the deltoid muscle.

NOTE: When properly placed, the combination of these two strips assists abduction.

14. Anchor the top of these last two strips with a strip of elastic adhesive tape.

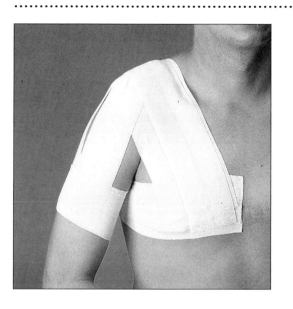

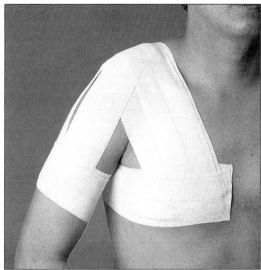

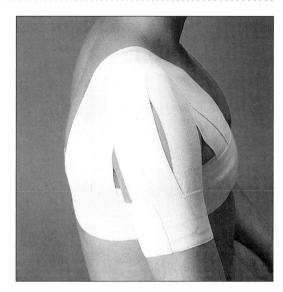

15. *Reapply the humeral (arm) anchor strip.*

16a. *Finish with a strip of elastic adhesive tape, applied as a horizontal anchor to the chest, to fix the lower ends of the vertical strips of tape.*

NOTE: Re-test sensation, pulse strength, temperature and colour ensuring that taping has not compromised circulation.

TIP: Place tensor wrap around chest for 10 minutes to ensure good adhesion.

16b. *Lateral view of finished taping.*
17. *Assess the degree of pain reduction post taping*
  a. *static*
  b. *with unassisted arm flexion and abduction*

TIP: For acute sprains, it also helps to support the weight of the forearm by adding a sling.

NOTE: The humeral (arm) portion of this tape job becomes optional several weeks post injury when unassisted arm movements are pain free without tape.

ANATOMICAL AREA: SHOULDER AND ELBOW

INJURY: SHOULDER SPRAIN ACROMIO-CLAVICULAR (A/C)
SEPARATION

T ERMINOLOGY:
- sprain of acromio-clavicular joint: 1st–3rd degree of severity. **(See sprains chart page 36).**
- shoulder separation

E TIOLOGY:
- direct impact to the point of the shoulder
- a fall; landing on the tip of the shoulder
- a severe fall on the outstretched arm
- common in hockey, rugby, football, horseback riding and martial arts.

S YMPTOMS:
- pain and tenderness over the top of the acromio-clavicular joint
- local swelling and bruising
- active movement testing: pain on all movements; particularly on flexion and horizontal adduction
- resistance testing: pain on all movements
- passive movement testing: pain on horizontal adduction
- stress testing: varying degrees of pain and step deformity between the clavicle and the acromion in 2nd and 3rd degrees of sprain severity.

T REATMENT:
Early:
- R.I.C.E.S.
- taped support: **for A/C Separation Taping page 176** a sling can offer additional support during first 48 hours
- therapeutic modalities
- 2nd and 3rd degree sprains should have at least three weeks of inactivity and support before dynamic treatment is started.

NOTE: Severe 3rd degree shoulder sprains may require surgery.

Later:
- continued physiotherapy including:
  - therapeutic modalities
  - range of motion and flexibility exercises
  - strengthening: isometric at first
  - carefully guided progressive functional strengthening as tolerated
- gradual return to pain-free sports activity with taped support: **A/C Separation Taping page 176.**
- a felt donut over the joint can further protect it from impact in contact sports.

NOTES:
- Premature return to activity risks further injury, escalating a 2nd degree sprain to a 3rd degree sprain (rupture).
- No muscles cross the A/C joint, therefore muscle strengthening does not specifically reinforce it.

S EQUELAE:
- instability
- chronic pain
- associated strain of deltoid or trapezius muscles can cause residual weakness
- arthritic changes: osteophyte formations
- "clicking"

R.I.C.E.S. : Rest, Ice, Compress, Elevate, Support

GLENO-HUMERAL (SHOULDER) DISLOCATION/SUBLUXATION TAPING:

Purpose:
- prevents elevation
- severely limits possible abduction external rotation and flexion of the shoulder
- allows relatively functional range of motion below the plane of 90°.

Indications for use:
- sub-acute shoulder subluxation
- chronic subluxation (anterior or inferior
- sub-acute shoulder dislocations
- apprehension in a previously or frequently injured athlete

This taping technique is not intended for an acute dislocation of the shoulder.

MATERIALS:

razor
skin toughener spray
7.5 cm (3 in.) elastic adhesive tape
3.8 cm (1.5 in.) white tape
gauze squares, prowrap, or felt

NOTES:
- Be certain that the correct diagnosis has been made in order to determine correct treatment:
- For repeat injuries check for possible axillary nerve damage: deltoid weakness (abduction at 90°) and lateral shoulder numbness
- Check that X-rays were taken after initial injury
- Check stability tests for different types of chronic subluxations/dislocations:

1. anterior
- positive "apprehension test" (muscle guarding when shoulder is passively externally rotated at 90° of abduction)
- anterior instability on the "load and shift test": excessive anterior gliding of the humeral head when pressed forward while stabilizing the scapula (athlete sitting)

2. inferior
- inferior instability: longitudinal traction causes an inferior displacement and a palpable sulcus (hollow) at the tip of the acromion (Athlete sitting or lying.)

3. posterior
- posterior instability or "clicking": when returning to a neutral position, after over-pressure is applied to a flexed and internally rotated shoulder (athlete sitting).
- posterior instability on the "load and shift test": excessive posterior gliding of the humeral head when pressed backwards while stabilizing the scapula (athlete sitting).
- Athletes who sustain repeat true dislocations should seek top orthopaedic advice, as this pathology can cause irreversible damage to the shoulder joint and surrounding structures.
- The female athlete can be taped using this technique, by applying the thoracic (chest) anchor below the breasts.
- Tender skin at the axilla (armpit) requires special care and protection.

For additional details regarding an injury example see TESTS chart page 190

Positioning:

Sitting, with hand resting comfortably on the ipsilateral (same side) thigh, and the elbow pointing sideways. This position keeps the shoulder in internal rotation. Ensure that the elbow does not fall backwards.

Procedure:

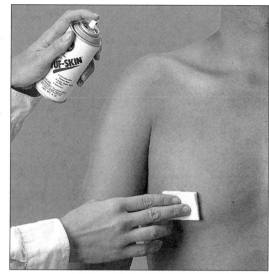

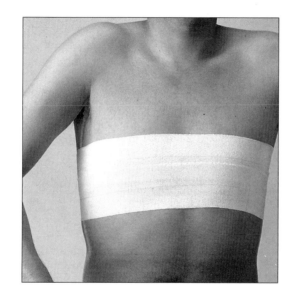

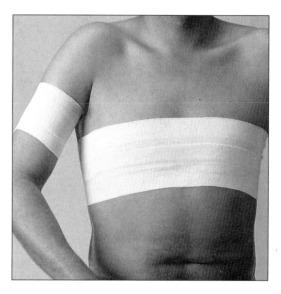

1. Wash and dry the skin, checking for cuts, abrasions or sensitive areas. Shave the upper humerus (arm) and chest area to be taped.

2. Apply skin toughener spray to minimize irritation and improve tape adherence.

TIP: Turn athlete's face away and protect the nipple when spraying.

NOTE: Check sensation, pulse, temperature and colour before starting to tape.

3. Cover the athlete's nipples with gauze, prowrap or felt.

4. Apply two circumferential strips 7.5 cm (3 in.) elastic adhesive tape around the thorax with moderate tension. (No tension over last 3 inches at each end in order to avoid peeling-back).

NOTE: For female athletes, apply this strip below breasts, raising up slightly laterally on injured side.

5. Apply two circumferential anchors of 7.5 (3 in.) elastic adhesive tape lightly around the mid-humerus (mid upper arm) at the distal end of the deltoid muscle.

Shoulder Dislocation

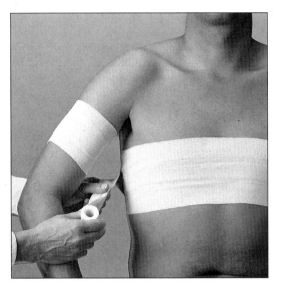

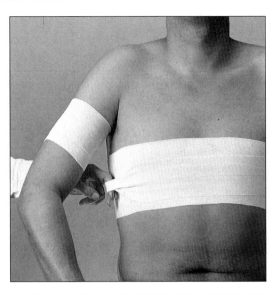

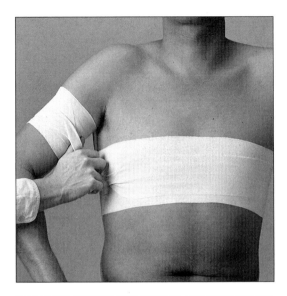

6. *With only moderate tension, wrap a circumferential strip of 7.5 cm (3 in.) elastic adhesive tape over the thoracic anchor:*

a. *Pinch it at the side,*

6b. *form a loop, and continue across the anterior chest wall.*

7. *Apply the same technique over the humeral (arm) anchor, forming a loop on the medial side.*

TIP: Ensure that the elbow points laterally, not posteriorly, and that the two loops face each other.

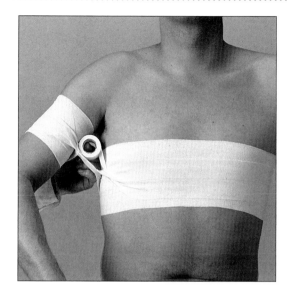

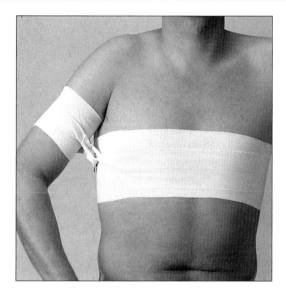

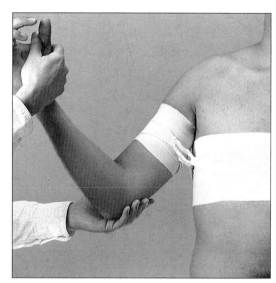

8a. *To form a check-rein, pass a small roll of 3 .8 cm (1.5 in.) tape through these loops.*

8b. *Attach them together to form a tether with 1.5 in. white tape.*

9. *The stability of the shoulder can be **cautiously** tested at this stage.*

TIP: Folding the white tape edges back, will ensure a stable unrippable tether.

NOTE: Recheck sensation, pulse, temperature and colour.

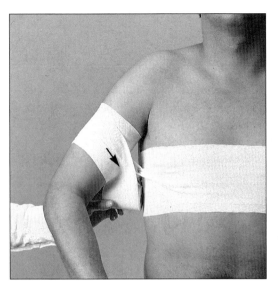

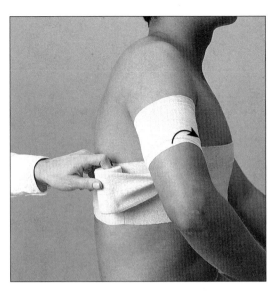

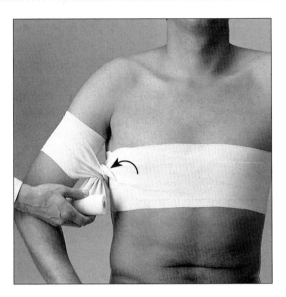

10. A figure-8 can now be applied with 7.5 cm (3 in.) elastic adhesive tape to ensure stability of the taping.

a. Begin on the lateral aspect of the humeral anchor, moving anteriorly.

10b. Pass between the humerus and the thorax, (arm and chest) rotating around the tether and continue along the posterior thoracic anchor.

10c. Bring the tape around the chest to the anterior side and twist the roll of tape around the tether.

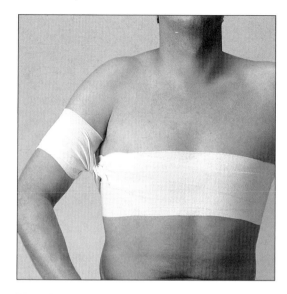

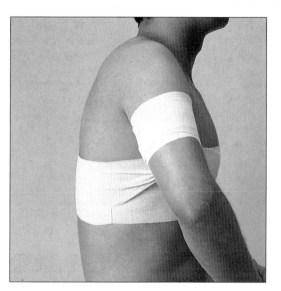

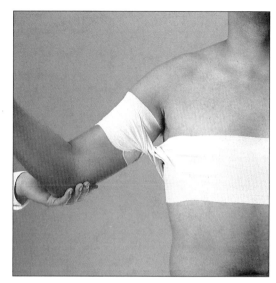

10d. Finish the figure-8, wrapping the strip around the humerus with minimal tension.

10e. View from the lateral side.

NOTE: Sensation, pulse strength, temperature and colour must be reassessed to ensure that the taping has not compromised circulation.

11. Test the degree of restriction:
- **a.** external notation must be limited to 30°
- **b.** abduction must be limited to 45°
- **c.** flexion must be limited
- **d.** the athelete must feel secure without any sense of apprehension on stress testing

ANATOMICAL AREA: SHOULDER AND ELBOW

INJURY: SHOULDER SPRAIN: GLENO-HUMERAL DISLOCATION

TERMINOLOGY:
- 3rd degree sprain of gleno-humeral joint.
- shoulder dislocation: anterior or posterior

ETIOLOGY:
- forced external rotation plus abduction of the shoulder in varying degrees of elevation or a direct blow to the posterior aspect of the shoulder usually cause an **anterior** dislocation (by far the most common type of dislocation).
- a fall on the tip outstretched hand or a direct blow or fall on the anterior aspect of the shoulder can cause a **posterior** dislocation.
- partial **anterior** dislocation (subluxation) is quite common in contact and collision sports, when the athlete's arm is caught out from the side (abduction) with the hand upwards (external rotation).
- chronic subluxations are common among athletes who perform repetitive movements at high speed at the outer reaches of their range of motion (such as baseball pitchers) or with great force (such as competitive swimmers).
- common injury in the following sports: hockey, football, basketball, baseball, wrestling, rugby, gymnastics.

SYMPTOMS:
- athlete feels shoulder has "popped out".
- a solid bulge either anteriorly or posteriorly
- hollow drop at tip of acromion
- active movement testing: extreme pain and inhibition of all movements
- resistance testing: (neutral position): pain in all directions
- inability to actively contract biceps and deltoid muscles
- passive movement testing: extreme pain on attempted passive internal or external rotation And abduction
- stress testing: **see introductory notes for Chronic Subluxations/Dislocations page 184.**

R.I.C.E.S. : Rest, Ice, Compress, Elevate, Support

> **NOTES:**
> - X-rays should be obtained in order to rule out possible fractures often associated with dislocations.
> - Watch for lateral shoulder-cap numbness or inability to contract the deltoid (resisted abduction): possible axillary nerve damage. This condition needs urgent attention and follow up

TREATMENT:
Early:
- R.I.C.E.S.
- reduction by an experienced professional
- immobilization: forearm should be strapped to chest wall for first three weeks before progressing to more dynamic treatment.
- therapeutic modalities

> **NOTES:**
> - Surgery is often indicated for extreme damage including avulsions, fractures, chips and nerve or vascular injury.

Later:
- continued physiotherapy including:
  - therapeutic modalities
  - isometric strengthening
  - progressive range of motion and flexibility exercise avoiding external rotation: (second 3 weeks)
- specific strengthening of internal rotators and adductors
- gradual return to activities with taped support: **Gleno-humeral taping page 184.**
- full rehabilitation program to regain strength and coordination: muscle stimulation or biofeedback are helpful.

SEQUELAE:
- recurrent dislocations
- permanently lax capsule
- weakness of shoulder rotators
- imbalance: abnormal coordination of shoulder girdle musculature
- arthritic changes

TAPING FOR ELBOW HYPEREXTENSION SPRAIN

Purpose:
- supports the elbow laterally
- limits the last 30° of extension and end-range pronation of the forearm
- allows full flexion and almost full supination

Indications for use:
- acute, sub-acute or chronic hyperextension sprains of the elbow
- posterior impingement syndrome
- medial sprains of the elbow, supported by reinforcing the medial **X** strips
- lateral sprains of the elbow, supported by reinforcing the lateral **X** strips
- combination ligament sprains
- chronic instability following fracture, dislocation of the elbow

MATERIALS:

razor
skin toughener spray
prowrap
5 cm (2 in.) elastic adhesive tape
7.5 cm (3 in.) elastic adhesive tape
3.8 cm (1.5 in.) white non-elastic adhesive tape
7.5 cm (3 in.) elastic wrap bandage

NOTES:
- Ensure a proper diagnosis by a sports medicine specialist.
- X-rays should be taken to rule out possibility of fracture.
- Pain or laxity on lateral stress testing with the elbow at 15° flexion, will indicate the need for added medial or lateral support
- Easily irritated structures include the biceps tendon, soft skin in elbow crease and the ulnar nerve or "funny bone", found posterio-mediality in the groove.
- If forearm anchor is too tight, circulation of the forearm will be constricted.

For additional details regarding an injury example see TESTS chart page 197.

Positioning

Sitting, with the elbow held in 40° flexion. The forearm should be in a neutral position between pronation and supination with the hand in a functional position.

Procedure:

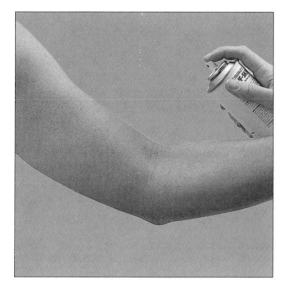
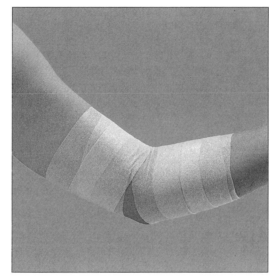
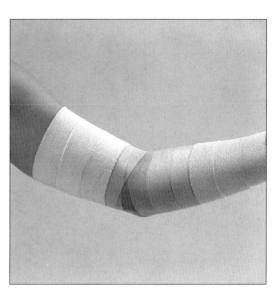

1. *Wash skin, dry, and check for cuts, abrasions or sensitive areas. Shave two (2) bands of skin (approximately 13 cm (5 in.) mid upper arm and mid to upper forearm.)*
2. *Spray the elbow up to and including the shaved bands of skin with skin toughener.*

NOTE: Sensation, pulse, temperature and colour of hand must be checked prior to taping.

3. *Apply prowrap from the proximal (upper) one-third of the forearm to the distal (lower) one-third of the humerus.*

NOTE: Padding and lubricant may be applied on the anterior aspect of the elbow to protect the biceps tendon and the soft skin when returning to sports with significant repetitive elbow motion.

4. *Apply 2 circumferential anchors of 5 cm (2 in.) elastic adhesive tape with minimal tension to the mid-humerus half-covering the prowrap and half-covering the skin directly.*
5. *Repeat 2 similar anchors mid to lower forearm.*

Elbow Sprain

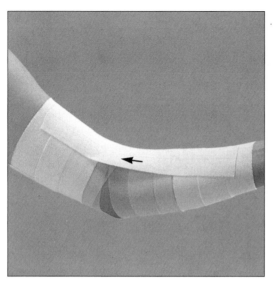

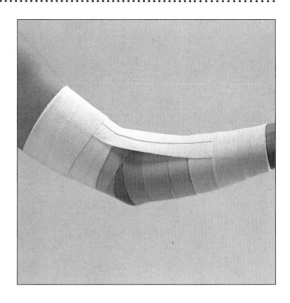

6. *To form a check-rein place the elbow in 45° of flexion and apply a vertical strip of 5 cm (2 in.) elastic adhesive tape from the lower anchor with tension to the upper anchor, directly over the anterior aspect of the elbow joint.*

7. *Repeat this strip overlapped by 1/2 the tape width more laterally.*

8. *Anchor these strips at both ends.*

TIP: Remember to keep the hand in a functional position.

TIP: Be certain to apply theses strips with enough tension to block the last 30° of extension when elbow is fully stretched.

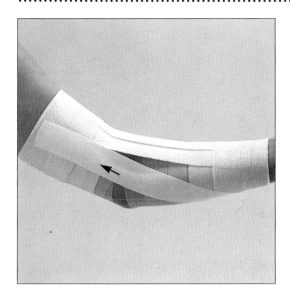 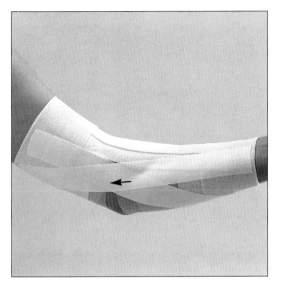 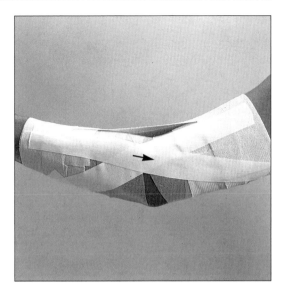

9. *For medial stability, hold the elbow bent at 35° of flexion, and apply a vertical strip of 3.8 cm (1.5 in.) white tape from the distal anchor to the upper anchor with strong tension.*

10. *Apply a second strip to form a **X** across the medial joint line of the elbow also with strong tension.*

NOTE: For medial sprains ensure a varus (inwardly bent) position and apply a second white tape "X" on the medial side with great tension.

11. *Repeat the white tape **X** on the lateral aspect to cross at the lateral joint line.*

NOTE: For lateral sprains ensure a more valgus (outwardly bent) position and apply a second white "X" on the lateral side with great tension.

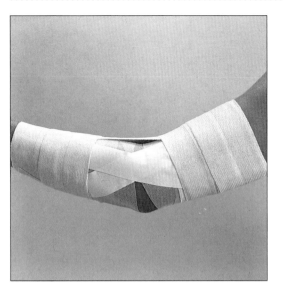

12a. *Apply two anchors distally and proximally using 7.5 cm (3 in.) elastic adhesive tape.*

NOTE: In closing up, a space is left at the anterior elbow, to avoid undue irritation to the sensitive underlying structures.

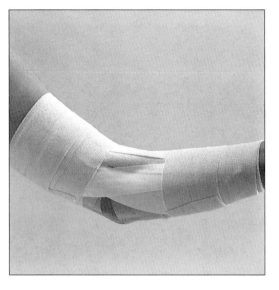

12b. *Anterior view of finishing taping.*

NOTE: Hand sensation, pulse, temperature and colour must be reassessed to ensure that taping has not compromised circulation.

13. *Test the degree of restriction:*
a. *extension should be limited by 30°or more.*
b. *there should be no pain on passive extension or lateral stress testing.*

TIP: Wrap the tape job with a 7.5 cm (3 in.) tensor bandage for 10 minutes to ensure good adherence.

ANATOMICAL AREA: SHOULDER AND ELBOW

INJURY: ELBOW SPRAIN: HYPEREXTENSION

T ERMINOLOGY:
- sprain of medial or lateral collateral ligaments (*see* **sprains chart page 36)**
- tearing of anterior joint capsule.

E TIOLOGY:
- fall on outstretched hand.
- forced hyperextension of the elbow (anterior capsule with/without medial and/or lateral ligament sprain.
- forced valgus (inward) stress causes damage to the medial collateral ligament (more vulnerable and more common).
- forced varus (outward) stress causes damage to the medial collateral ligament.
- chronic medial sprains are common in pitchers and javelin throwers

S YMPTOMS:
- pain on anterior capsule – medial and/or lateral joint line – implies localized injury site
- swelling
- active movement testing: pain on end-range extension
- resistance testing: (neutral position):
  a. no significant pain on moderate resistance
  b. pain on flexion if biceps simultaneously injured
- stress testing: varying degrees of pain and laxity on stress testing (done at 15° flexion). Amount of laxity indicates degree of injury. (*see* **Notes page 192.)**

> NOTES: Any suspicion of deformity requires immediate medical attention and X-rays.

T REATMENT:
Early:
- R.I.C.E.S.
- sling
- therapeutic modalities

Later:
- continued physiotherapy including:
  - therapeutic modalities
  - taping for limited activity: **for Elbow hyperextension taping see page 192.**
    - gentle traction and mobilization
- progressive resistance rehabilitation program for humero-ulnar as well as radio-ulnar joints.
- gradual return to activities with taped support as above.

S EQUELAE:
- chronic instability
- ulnar nerve paraesthesia
- adhesions causing reduced range of motion
- arthritic changes
- calcification of ligaments

Elbow Sprain

R.I.C.E.S. : Rest, Ice, Compress, Elevate, Support

Notes

Chapter Nine ....

WRIST AND HAND

The **wrist** is a pliable osteo-ligamentous complex forming a connecting link between the forearm and the hand. Multi-directional mobility results from the numerous multi-articular carpal bones which, along with the radio-ulnar joints, allow the hand to be positioned functionally at any angle. Stability is derived from the complex array of ligaments often injured when falling on an outstretched hand. Vascular supply to the carpal bones is often compromised with ligamentous damage.

The **hand**, while being the most active and intricate joint complex in the body, is the least protected. Constructed as a series of complex, delicately balanced joints, it offers manipulating ability, dexterity and precision. This highly sensitive structure used to hold, hit, catch and manipulate, is particularly vulnerable to trauma when subjected to repetitive stresses or the impact of falls.

Providing adequate support while still maintaining functional movement is the prime consideration when taping the hand and/or wrist.

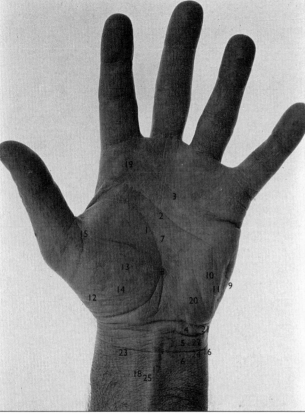

Palm of the left hand

The surface markings of various structures within the wrist and hand are indicated, not all of them are palpable, e.g. the superficial and deep palmar arches (7,8), but their relative positions are important

- The curved lines proximal to the base of the fingers indicate the ends of the head of the metacarpophalangeal joints.
- The creases on the fingers indicate the level of the interphalangeal joints.
- The middle crease at the wrist indicates the level of the wrist joint.
- The radial artery at the wrist (23) is the commonest site for feeling the pulse. The vessel is on the radial side of the tendon of flexor carpi radialis (18) and can be compressed against the lower end of the radius.
- The median nerve at the wrist (25) lies on the ulnar side of the tendon of flexor carpi radialis (18) and is absent in percent of limbs).
- The ulnar nerve and artery at the wrist (22, 23) are on the radial side of the tendon of flexor carpi ulnaris (16) and the pisiform bone (21). The artery is on the radial side of the nerve and its pulsation can be felt, though less easily than that of the radial artery (23).
- Abductor pollicis brevis (12) and flexor pollicis brevis (13) together with the underlying opponents pollicis, are the muscles which form the thenar eminence, the 'bulge' at the base of the thumb. Abductor digiti minimi (9) and flexor digiti minimi brevis (10), together with the underlying opponens digiti minimi, form the muscles of the hypothenar eminence, the less prominent bulge on the ulnar side of the palm where palmaris brevis (11) lies subcutaneously.

CREASES	MUSCLES	TENDONS	ARTERIES
1 LONGITUDINAL	9 ABDUCTOR DIGITI MINIMI	16 FLEXOR CARPI ULNARIS	22 ULNAR
2 PROXIMAL TRANSVERSE	10 FLEXOR DIGITI MINIMUS	17 PALMARIS LONGUS BREVIS	23 RADIAL
3 DISTAL TRANSVERSE	11 PALMARIS BREVIS	18 FLEXOR CARPI RADIALIS	**NERVES**
4 DISTAL WRIST	12 ABDUCTOR POLLICIS	**BREVIS BONES**	24 ULNAR
5 MIDDLE WRIST	13 FLEXOR POLLICIS BREVIS	19 HEAD OF METACARPAL	25 MEDIAN
6 PROXIMAL WRIST	14 THENOR EMINENCE	20 HOOK OF HAMATE	
ARCHES	15 ADDUCTOR POLLICIS	21 PISIFORM	
7 SUPERFICIAL PALMAR			
8 DEEP PALMAR			

SURFACE ANATOMY

Dorsum of the left hand

The fingers are extended at the metacarpo-phalangeal joints, causing the extensor tendons of the fingers (1, 2 and 3) to stand out, and partially flexed at the interphalangeal joints.

The thumb is extended at the carpometacarpal joint and partially flexed at the metacarpophalangeal and interphalangeal joints. The lines proximal to the bases of the fingers indicate the ends of the heads of the metacarpophalangeal joints. The anatomical snuffbox (9) is the hollow between the tendons of abductor pollicis longus (7) and extensor pollicis brevis (6) laterally and extensor pollicis longus medially (5).

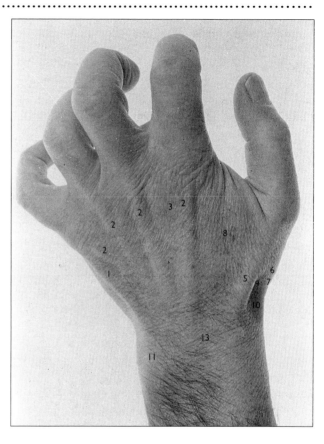

TENDONS	BONES
1 EXTENSOR DIGITI MINIMI	9 ANATOMICAL SNUFF BOX OVER SCAPHOID
2 EXTENSOR DIGITORUM	10 STYLOID PROCESS OF RADIUS
3 EXTENSOR INDICIS	11 HEAD OF ULNA
4 EXTENSOR CARPI RADIALIS LONGUS	**VEINS**
5 EXTENSOR POLLICIS LONGUS	12 CEPHALIC
6 EXTENSOR POLLICIS BREVIS	**RETINACULUM**
7 ABDUCTOR POLLICIS LONGUS	13 EXTENSOR RETINACULUM
MUSCLES	
8 FIRST DORSAL INTEROSSEUS	

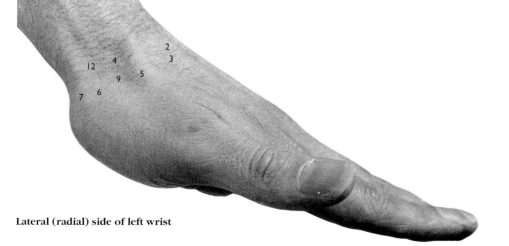

Lateral (radial) side of left wrist

WRIST HYPEREXTENSION SPRAIN TAPING:

Purpose:
- reinforces the collateral ligaments of the wrist and the anterior joint structures
- restricts extension and limits the last degrees of radial and ulnar deviation (sideways movement)
- permits functional use of the hand.

Indications for use:
- palmar radio-carpal ligament (wrist hyperextension) sprains
- for dorsal radio-carpal ligament (wrist hyperflexion) sprains: apply the check-rein dorsally (back of wrist) and add restraining **X**'s to the dorsal aspect of the wrist thus limiting end-range flexion
- for radial collateral ligament sprain: reinforce the lateral **X** and add a lateral palmar **X** to prevent ulnar deviation
- for ulnar collateral ligament sprain: reinforce the medial **X** and add a medial palmar **X** to prevent radial deviation
- diffuse pain in the wrist due to repeated compression, or "jamming" the wrist
- wrist pain post-immobilization.

MATERIALS:

razor
skin toughener spray
prowrap
3.8 cm (1.5 in.) white tape

NOTES:
- Ensure that a proper diagnosis has been made to rule out fractures - particularly if the injury was caused by a fall on the outstretched hand. (The scaphiod bone [first carpal bone at the base of the thumb] is the most commonly fractured.)
- Clarify the mechanism of injury, whether it was hyperextension or hyperflexion that occurred.
- The use of skin toughener or quick dry adhesive spray is essential for adherence of taping, especially in rainy or hot conditions when hands, wrists and forearms tend to become quite damp.
- Wrap the circumferential strips with minimal tension, to avoid neurovascular compromise.
- Monitor circulatory status and sensation prior to, during and after taping.

For additional details regarding an injury example see TESTS chart page 206.

Positioning:

Sitting, with the wrist in a neutral position held in slight extension (approximately 20°).

> TIP: The elbow can be supported on a table for added stability. (Not shown in photos.)

Procedure:

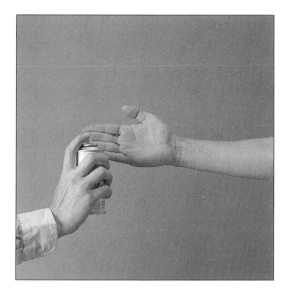 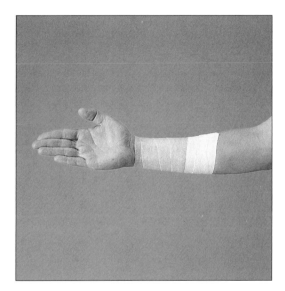 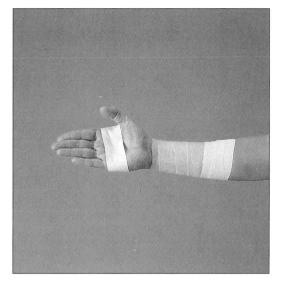

1. Wash, dry and shave the forearm, if hairy. Check for cuts, abrasions and sensitive skin.
2. Spray the area to be taped.

3. Apply prowrap to the forearm.
4. Apply 2 circumferential anchors of 3.8 cm (1.5 in.) white tape around mid-forearm at the musculotendinous junction, following the soft tissue contours.

5. Apply a circumferential anchor of white tape around the distal metacarpals (palm of hand)

> TIP: Ensure that these anchors do not unduly restrict splaying of the metacarpals.

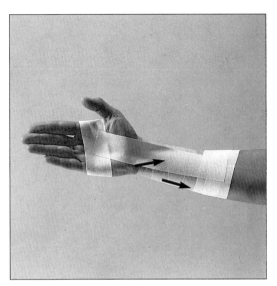

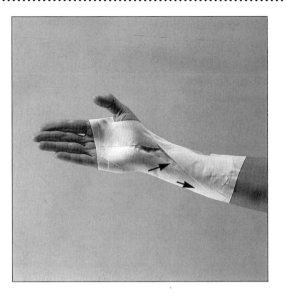

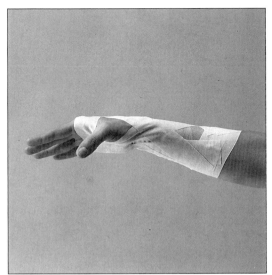

6. *Hold the wrist at 0° extension and apply a check-rein (restraining strip) from the anterior aspect of the distal anchor to the proximal, with strong tension, passing across the anterior joint line.*

NOTE: A second check-rein can be added, overlapping the first by 1/2 for added strength and/or for wide wrists (not illustrated)

7. *Start the medial **X** from the anterior aspect of the distal anchor to the posterio-medial aspect of the proximal anchor.*

8. *Finish this **X** with a strip from the posterio-medial aspect of the distal anchor to the proximal anchor anteriorly with firm tension.*

NOTE: The X formed by these two strips should cross on the anterio-medial joint line.

9. *Begin a lateral **X** with a strip from the posterior aspect of the distal anchor pulling with tension to the anterior aspect of the proximal anchor.*

10. *Finish this **X** with a strip from the anterior aspect of the distal anchor to the lateral aspect of the proximal anchor.*

NOTE: The X formed by these two strips should cross on the anterio-lateral joint line.

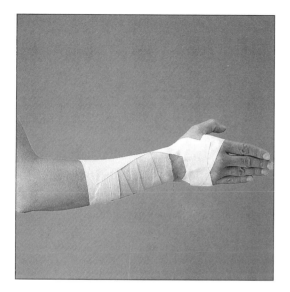

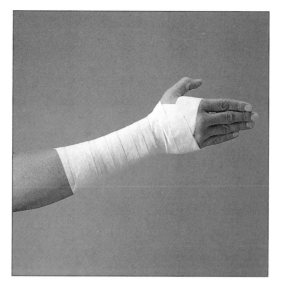

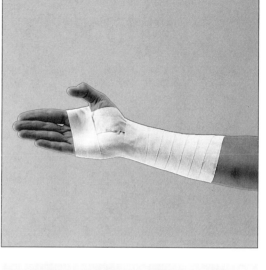

11. *Reanchor these supporting* **X**s *both distally and proximally.*

NOTE: For added stability, posterior Xs can be added at this time, holding the wrist 20°or less of extension. (Not shown in photos).

12. *Close up the hand portion of the taping by overlapping the distal anchor by a half-width of the next circumferential strip of white tape.*

13. *Continue closing up the tape job with overlapping light circumferential strips.*

14. *Test the degree of restriction: extension should be limited to 30° or less. There must be no pain on passive extension at the wrist..*

NOTE: Check finger colour and sensation for signs of compromised circulation.

Wrist Sprain

ANATOMICAL AREA: WRIST AND HAND

IINJURY: WRIST HYPEREXTENSION SPRAIN

T ERMINOLOGY:
- partial or complete tearing of anterior wrist capsule
- partial or complete tearing of radial and/or ulnar collateral ligaments. **See Sprains chart page 36.**

E TIOLOGY:
- fall on outstretched hand
- forced hyperextension during a tackle with an opponent
- overloaded weight-lifting

S YMPTOMS:
- pain over anterior joint capsule and ligaments
- decreased range of motion
- swelling
- active movement testing: pain on end-range exrension
- passive movement testing:
  a. pain on exention
  b. pain posssible on end-range flexion resulting from compression of injured tissues
- resistance testing (neutral position): no significant pain with moderate resistance; pain possible on flexion if flexors also involved
- stress testing: varying degrees of pain and laxity

> NOTE: If wrist is unstable when testing ligaments, X-rays must be taken to rule out the possibility of fracture.

T REATMENT:
Early:
- R.I.C.E.S.
- initially: elastic tensor compression and sling support with careful attention to circulation for the first 48 hours
- therapeutic modalities, contrast baths

Later:
- continued physiotherapy including:
  - therapeutic modalities
  - flexibility exercises
  - strengthening (isometric initially)
- total rehabilitation program for mobility, flexibility, strengthening and dexterity
- taping for gradual return to pain-free functional activities. **For Wrist Taping *see* page 202.**

> NOTE: Sprains that do not resond well to treatment should be reassessed by a hand specialist. Pain and clicking on the ulnar side may imply damage to the triangular fibro-catilage (meniscus). Persistent pain on the radial side may indicate a necrosis or missed fracture of the scaphoid (circulation of the carpal bones often compromised with wrist sprains)

S EQUELAE:
- tenosynovitis
- weakness
- chronic sprain
- instability
- degenerative joint changes
- stubborn cases may suggest an associated meniscal tear and require some form of splinting for dunamic activity

R.I.C.E.S. : Rest, Ice, Compress, Elevate, Support

Notes

THUMB SPRAIN TAPING:

Purpose:
- supports the collateral ligaments of the first metacarpal phalangeal joint
- prevents the last degrees of extension, limits abduction
- allows some flexion
- does not compromise wrist and hand function

Indications for use:
- metacarpo-phalangeal joint (MCPJ) sprain (ulnar ligament)
- carpometacarpal joint (CMCJ) sprain (ulnar aspect); reinforce the diagonal anchor
- skier's thumb, "gamekeeper's" thumb
- post-immobilization tenderness
- post-surgery of 3rd degree repair

MATERIALS:

razor
skin toughener spray
prowrap
3.8 cm (1.5 in.) white tape
1.2 cm (0.5in.) white tape

NOTES:
- If a 3rd degree sprain be suspected (greater that 35°of passive adduction) a hand surgeon should be seen as early as possible.
- X-rays will rule out the possibility of an avulsion fracture.
- Thoroughly inspect the hand for cuts, abrasions and any other possible sources of infection.
- Watch carefully for signs of restricted circulation - particularly during the first 48 hours post-injury when swelling tends to be greatest.
- Restricted circulation, apart from causing discomfort, can be particularly dangerous in below-freezing weather (increased risk of frostbite)
- Hand and thumb size will dictate the width of tape required.

For additional details regarding an injury example see TESTS chart page 214.

Positioning:

Sitting with the elbow supported on a table, the thumb and hand held in a neutral, functional position.

Procedure:

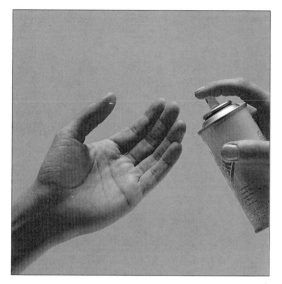

1. Wash, dry and spray the area to be taped.

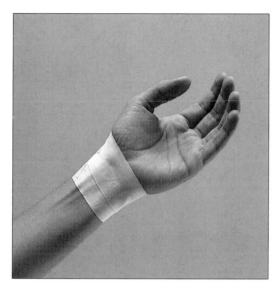

2. Apply two circumferential strips of 3.8 cm (1.5 in.) white tape around the wrist using light tension.

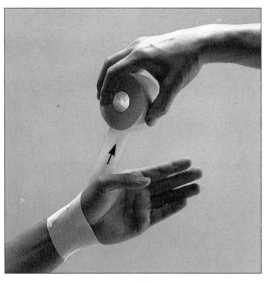

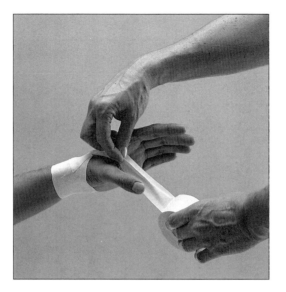

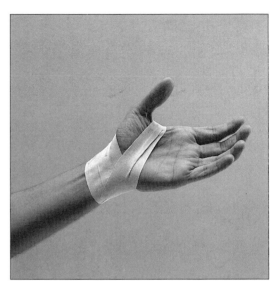

3. *Apply the distal anchor:*

a. *Using 3.8 cm (1.5 in) white tape, start from the posterior side of the proximal anchor, wrap around the wrist, pull up and across the dorsum of the hand.*

3b. *Cross from posterior to anterior between the thumb and index finger.*

c. *Pinch the tape as it passes through the web space, to narrow the tape and to avoid irritating the soft skin at this site.*

TIP: Be careful not to apply any pressure through the web space.

3d. *Continue diagonally across the palmar aspect of the hand and fix the strip medially on the proximal anchor.*

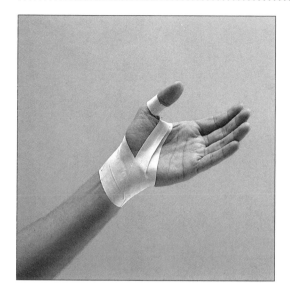

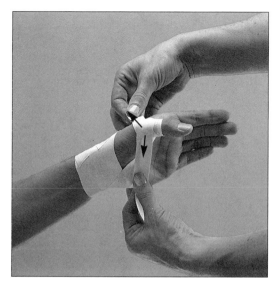

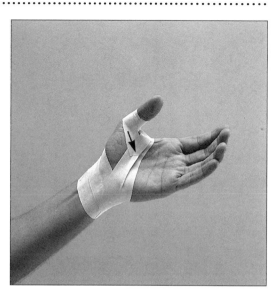

4. *Apply the thumb anchor lightly, placing the strip circumferentially around the proximal phalanx following its contours.*

5. *Apply an incomplete figure-8 strip of 1.2 cm (0.5 in.) white tape by pulling gently around the thumb, crossing the strips and pulling equally with both hands medially, adducting the thumb before adhering both ends of this strip to the anchor.*

6. *The anterior end is applied to the palmar anchor, and the posterior end is applied to the dorsal anchor with firm pressure.*

TIP: Be careful not to apply strong pressure circumferentially around the thumb during application of tape.

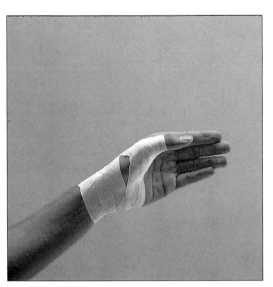

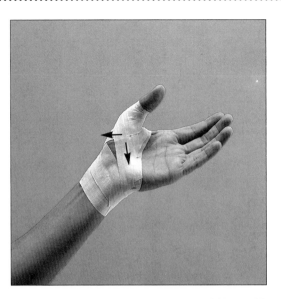

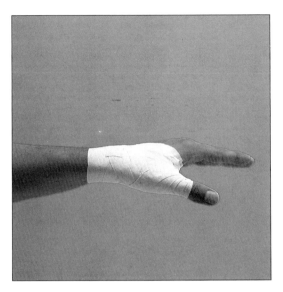

7a. *Apply another half-figure-8 more proximally overlapping by 2/3 the width of the tape on the thumb anchor.*

7b. *Allow the strip ends fan out slightly as they reach the anchor.*

8. *Continue repeating the half-figure-8s overlapping by 1/2 to 2/3 the width of the tape, moving proximally down the thumb.*

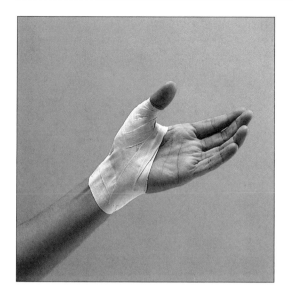

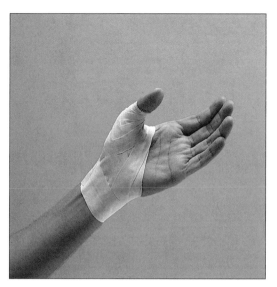

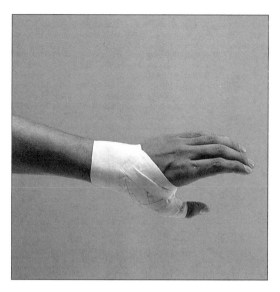

9. *Re-anchor the ends of the incomplete figure-8s with another diagonal anchor.*

TIP: Be careful not to apply strong pressure through the web space.

NOTE: A figure-8 check-rein can be applied between the thumb and first finger to further restrict abduction. (Not shown in photos.)

10. *Apply circumferential strips of 3.8 cm (1.5 in.) white tape around the wrist covering the diagonal anchor and any remaining tape ends.*

11. *Check functional position of the hand and test the degree of restriction: extension and abduction must be limited by 20° or more. There should be no pain on passive movements of the thumb particularly extension and abduction.*

NOTE: Check thumb colour and sensation for signs of compromised circulation.

ANATOMICAL AREA: WRIST AND HAND

INJURY: THUMB SPRAIN

T ERMINOLOGY:
- partial or complete tearing of ulnar collateral ligament: the first MCPJ (metacarpal phalangeal joint); degree of severity 1st–3rd **(See SPRAINS Chart page 36).**
- "game-keeper's thumb"
- "skier's thumb"

E TIOLOGY:
- forced extension and/or abduction of the metacarpal-phalangeal joint
- a fall on an outstretched hand
- common in skiing

S YMPTOMS:
- tenderness over medial aspect of metacarpal-phalangeal joint (base of thumb in the web space)
- local swelling and/or discolouration
- active movement testing: pain on end-range extension
- passive movement testing: pain on extension plus abduction
- resistance testing: (neutral position): no significant pain on moderate resistance
- stress testing: more than 35° lateral of laxity in both flexion and extension indicates a complete rupture or an avulsion fracture.

T REATMENT:
Early:
- R.I.C.E.S. for first 48 hours
- therapeutic modalities; contrast baths
- range of motion (ROM) exercises
- taping: **for Thumb Sprain Taping see page 208.**

> NOTE: 3rd degree and severe 2nd degree require spica splinting, casting or surgery with at least 3 weeks of immobilization.

Later:
- continued physiotherapy including:
  - therapeutic modalities
  - joint mobilizations if stiff post-immobilization
  - strengthening (isometric at first)
- gradual return to pain-free functional activities with taped support: **(for Thumb Sprain taping, see page 208).**
- complete rehabilitation program including range of motion, flexibility, strengthening and dexterity

S EQUELAE:
- chronic instability with severe dysfunction
- weakness of grip
- tenosynovitis
- degenerative changes of metacarpal-phalangeal joint

R.I.C.E.S. : Rest, Ice, Compress, Elevate, Support

Notes

FINGER SPRAIN TAPING

MATERIALS:
razor
skin toughener spray
1.2 cm (0.5 in.) white tape

Purpose:
- supports the palmar and collateral ligaments of the finger
- prevents full extension
- allows full flexion

Indications for use:
- palmar ligament sprain (hypertextension) of the finger
- post-immobilization painful stiffness of the finger
- "jammed" or "stubbed" finger
- medial collateral ligament (MCL) sprain of the finger: reinforce medial **X**
- lateral collateral ligament (LCL) sprain of the finger reinforce lateral **X**

NOTES:
- Never allow the athlete to continue playing (even when taped), if a serious injury is suspected.
- Ensure a correct diagnosis by a sports-medicine or hand specialist. (Fractures and dislocations are often misdiagnosed and mistreated.)
- Localize the exact site of the injury: which aspect of which joint of which finger, and re-test for pain through range during and after the tape job is completed.
- Taping the injured finger to its neighbour ("buddy taping") further protects the injured ligaments while allowing function and movement.
- If the athlete needs to use the injured hand to handle a ball during a game, "buddy-tape" the fingers slightly apart to allow better control of the ball.

For additional details regarding an injury example see TESTS chart page 220.

Positioning:

Sitting with the elbow supported on a table and the finger(s) placed in a neutral, functional position. (Approximately 20° flexion.)

Procedure:

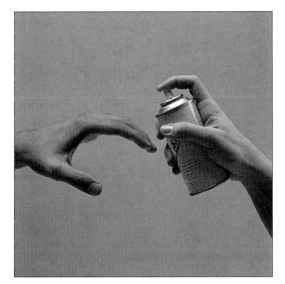

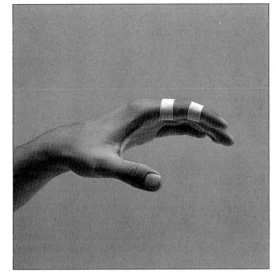

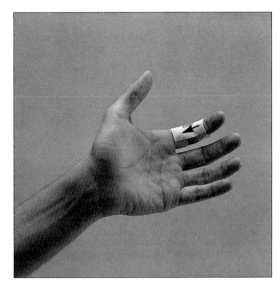

1. *Wash and dry finger, watching for cuts or abrasions.*
2. *Spray the area with skin toughener or adhesive spray.*

TIP: A cotton-tip applicator can be used to minimize the adherence of non-affected digits.

3. *Gently apply two circumferential anchors of 1.2 cm (0.5 in.) white tape, one above and one below the injured joint.*

TIP: Be careful to avoid constriction.

4. *Apply a vertical strip of 1.2 cm (0.5 in.) white tape from the distal anchor to the proximal anchor on the centre of the vular (under) aspect of the finger, with strong tension, keeping the finger flexed about 20°.*

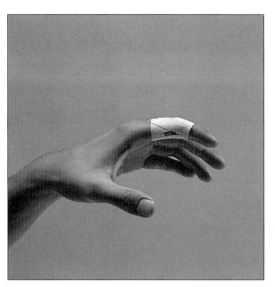

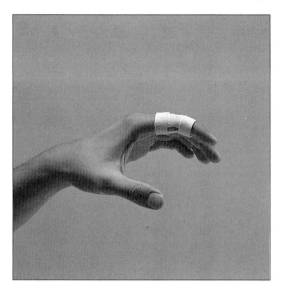

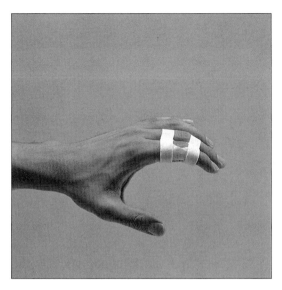

5. *Apply a lateral **X** with two strips from the distal anchor to the proximinal, with strong tension, forming the **X** on the lateral joint line.*

6. *Repeat the above on the medial aspect, with the **X** lying on the medial joint line.*

7. *Repeat the anchors as in **Step 2**, to cover the ends of the vertical strips.*

8. *Perform a simple "buddy-taping" technique by taping the injured finger to its neighbour.*

NOTE: This step is useful for sports not needing full hand function (as in soccer), when the fingers can function as a unit.

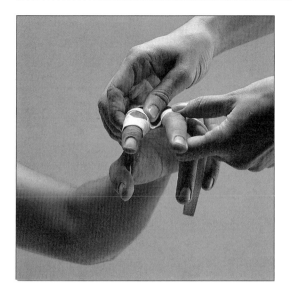 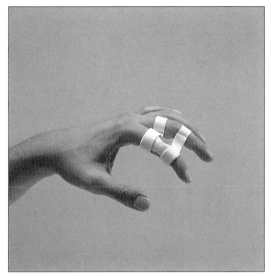 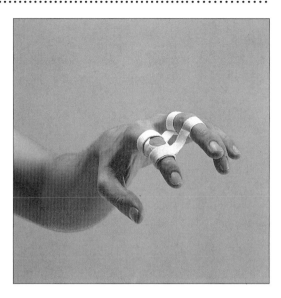

9. ***Alternative method:*** *apply a webbed "buddy-taping" by keeping the injured digit slightly abducted (spread apart) while taping it to its neighbour.*

NOTE: This technique is useful for sports requiring full functional dexterity and use of individual fingers (as in basketball or volleyball). Note that more space is left between the fingers with this option.

10. *Pinch the buddy tape strip between the fingers to allow some independent movement of the injured digit.*

11. *Check for functional dexterity and verify adequate limits of taping.*

NOTE: Finger colour and sensation must be checked for signs of compromised circulation.

12. *Test the degree of restriction: extension must be limited by 10° or more and there should be no pain on stressing the injured ligament.*

ANATOMICAL AREA: WRIST AND HAND

INJURY: FINGER SPRAIN

TERMINOLOGY:
- partial or complete rupture of palmar ligament (anterior capsule), medial collateral (ulnar) ligament or lateral collateral (radial) ligaments: degree of severity: 1st–3rd, **(See SPRAINS Chart page 36).**
- "stoved" finger
- "jammed" finger

E TIOLOGY:
- telescoping blow: direct compressive force on the tip of the finger (i.e. jamming it against a ball as in basketball or volleyball)
- torsional stresses
- sideways stress to a finger: may catch on clothing, equipment or terrain
- hyperextension of finger
- contusion of ligaments

S YMPTOMS:
- pain over site of injury
- swelling and discolouration
- local tenderness
- active movement testing: pain on end-range extension and/or flexion (pinching the injured capsule)
- passive movement testing: pain on end range extension and/or possibly on flexion
- resistance testing: (neutral position): no significant pain on moderate resistance
- stress testing:
  a. pain with or without laxity on lateral stress testing in 1st and 2nd degree sprains
  b. instability with 3rd degree sprains (often with less pain).

T REATMENT:
Early:
- R.I.C.E.S.
- initial taping: loose **Buddy Taping page 218.**
- therapeutic modalities; contrast baths
- range of motion exercises

NOTE: 3rd degree and severe 2nd degree sprains usually require splinting with at least one week of complete immobilization and 2 weeks of mobilization between treatments and range of motion (ROM) exercises, followed by eight (8) weeks of taped support.

Later:
- continued physiotherapy including:
  - therapeutic modalities
  - mobilizations
  - flexibility
- strengthening exercises for all hand musculature.
- taping for gradual return to pain-free functional activities. **For Thumb Sprain taping,** *see* **page 216.**
- progressive exercises for range of motion strength and dexterity.

S EQUELAE:
- persistent laxity (instability)
- chronic sprain reinjury
- deformity
- stiffness
- degenerative joint changes

R.I.C.E.S. : Rest, Ice, Compress, Elevate, Support

GLOSSARY

Anchor	Anything which makes stable or secure, anything which is depended upon for support or security.
Basketweave	An interlocking of two or more strands resembling a basket.
Bursa	A pouch or sacklike cavity containing synovia, located at points of friction.
Butterfly	A combination of taping strips with a typical form of wider top and bottom, and narrower middle.
Buttress	A prop or support used to strengthen a structure.
Capsule	A fibrous container that envelops some structure of the body, as in a joint.
Cartilage	A tough, elastic form of connective tissue found on articulating boney spaces.
Caudal	Of, or pertaining to the tail or posterior part of the body, opposed to cranial.
Cranial	Of, or pertaining to the skull or superior part of the body, opposed to caudal.
Distal	Relatively remote from the centre of the body or point of attachment, opposed to proximal.
Figure-8	A manouever that consists in tracing the figure "8".
Horizontal strip	A strip which is placed level with the horizon, opposed to vertical strip.
Horseshoe	Padding made to resemble the "U" shape of a horseshoe.
Inferior	Situated below or downward, opposed to superior.
Lateral	Situated at or relatively near the outer side of the point of reference, opposed to medial.
Ligament	A band of firm fibrous connective tissue forming a connection between bones offering stability.
Lock	Any part that fastens, secures or holds something firmly in place.
Medial	Situated at or relatively near the middle of the point of reference, opposed to lateral.
Plantar	Pertaining to the sole of the foot.
Proximal	Relatively near the central position of the body, opposed to distal.

GLOSSARY

Stirrup	Any "U"-shaped loop or piece.
Superior	Situated above or over another body part, opposed to inferior.
Tendon	A cord of tough elastic connective tissue formed at the termination of a muscle serving to transmit its force across a joint.
Vertical strip	A strip that is placed perpendicular to the line of the horizon, opposed to horizontal strip.
Valgus	Deformities which displace the distal part of a joint away from the midline.
Varus	Deformities which displace the distal part of the joint towards the midline.
Volar	Pertaining to the palm of the hand.

Glossary

REFERENCES ....

1. American Medical Association, *Standard Nomenclature of Athletic Injuries* A.M.A., Chicago, USA, 1966.

2. Austin, Karin, A., B.Sc.P.T., *Taping Booklet.* Physiothérapie International, Montreal, Canada, 1977.

3. Avis, Walter S., Editor, *Funk & Wagnalls Standard College Dictionary.* Fitzhenry & Whiteside Ltd., Toronto, Canada, 1978.

4[†] Backhouse, Kenneth M., O.B.E., V.R.D., and Hutchings R.T., *A Colour Atlas if Surface Anatomy.* Wolfe Medical Publications, London, UK, 1986.

5. Bouchard, Fernand, B.Sc. *Guide du soigneur.* Projet Perspective-Jeunesse, Montreal, Canada, 1972.

6. British Columbia Sports Medical Council, *British Columbia Sports Aid Program*, Victoria, B.C. Canada, 1984.

7. Cerney, J.V. M.D. *Complete Book of Athletic Taping Techniques*, Parker, New York, USA, 1972.

8. Cyriax, James, *Textbook of Orthopaedic Medical Diagnosis of Soft Tissue Injuries.* 8th Edition, Bailliere, Tindall, London, U.K, 1982

9. Dixon, Dwayne "Spike", A.T., *The Dixonary of Athletic Training.* Bloomcraft-Central Printing Inc., Bloomington, Indiana, USA, 1965.

10. Dominquez, Richard H., M.D., *The Complete Book of Sports Medicine.* Warner Books Inc., New York, USA. 1979.

11. Griffith, H. Winter, M.D., *Complete Guide to Sports Injuries.* The Body Press, HP Books Inc., Tucson, Arizona, USA, 1986.

12. Head, William F., M.S.F., *Treatment of Athletic Injuries.* Frank W. Horner Ltd.; Montreal, Canada, 1966.

13. Hess, Heinrich, Prof.., *Sportverletzungen.* Luitpold-Werk, München (Munich), Germany, 1984.

14. Kapandji, I.A., *The Physiology of the Joints Vol 1 & 2*, Churchill Livingstone Edinburgh, Scotland, 1970.

15. Logan, Gene A. Ph.D. R.P.T., and Logan Roland F., *Techniques of Athletic Training.* Franklin-Adams Press, Pasadena, California, USA. 1959.

16* Magee, David J. Orthopaedic *Physical Assessment*, Saunders, Philadelphia, USA. 1987.

17* McConnell, J., B.App.Sc.(Phtg)., Grad.Dip., *The Management of Chrondromalacia Patellae: a long-term solution*, Physiotherapy, 32, (4), 1986, 215-223.

18[†] McMinn, R.M.H., and Hutchings R.T., *A Colour Atlas of Human Anatomy.* Wolfe Publications, London, UK, 1977.

19[†] McMinn, R.M.H., Hutchings R.T and Logan B.M. *A Colour Atlas of Foot and Ankle Anatomy.* Wolfe Medical Publications, London, UK, 1982

20. Montag, Hans-Jürgen and Asmussen Peter D., *Functional Bandaging: A manual of bandaging technique.* Beiersdorf Bibliothek, Hamburg, Germany, 1981.

21* Reid, David C., *Sports Injury Assessment and Rehabilitation*, Churchill Livingstone, New York, USA, 1992.

22. Williams, Warwick (ed.) *Gray's Anatomy.* Churchill Livingstone Edinburgh, Scotland, 1970.

† Sources of our anatomy sections

* *Recommended reading*

T.E.S.T.S. Chart Listings

···

224

INDEX ....

therapeutic care, 22
thigh
  adductor strain, 166-70
  quadriceps contusion/strain, 158-64
thumb
  post-immobilization tenderness, 208
  sprain taping, 208-14
tibialis posterior
  support strips, 115
  tendinitis, 129
  tendon injury, 126-8
tissue repair, 22
toe sprain, 52-5, 56
turf toe, 52, 56

U

ulnar ligament sprain (thumb), 208
  collateral, 202

V

V-lock strip, 89, 92-3

W

welling, 22
white zinc oxide tape, 12, 18
wrist, 199
  compression, 202
  hyperextension sprain, 202-6
  hyperflexion, 202
  pain, 202, 205, 206